MULTIMODAL MANAGEMENT OF CANINE OSTEOARTHRITIS

SECOND EDITION

MULTIMODAL MANAGEMENT OF CANINE OSTEOARTHRITIS

SECOND EDITION

STEVEN M. FOX MS, DVM, MBA, PhD

Surgical Specialist: New Zealand VMA
President: Securos Surgical, A Division of AmerisourceBurgen
Independent Consultant, Clive, Iowa, USA
Adjunct Professor, College of Veterinary Medicine, University of Illinois
Adjunct Professor, Massey University, Palmerston North, New Zealand
Program Chairman (2000-02), President (2004), Veterinary Orthopedic Society

Special Section on Regenerative Medicine by

Brittany Jean Carr, DVM, CCRT & **Sherman O. Canapp,** DVM, MS,
CCRT Diplomate ACVS, Diplomate ACVSMR
Veterinary Orthopedic Sports Medicine Group, Annapolis Junction MD

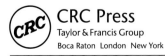

CRC Press
Taylor & Francis Group
Boca Raton London New York

CRC Press is an imprint of the
Taylor & Francis Group, an **informa** business

CRC Press
Taylor & Francis Group
6000 Broken Sound Parkway NW, Suite 300
Boca Raton, FL 33487-2742

© 2017 by Taylor & Francis Group, LLC
CRC Press is an imprint of Taylor & Francis Group, an Informa business

No claim to original U.S. Government works

Printed and bound in India by Replika Press Pvt. Ltd.

Printed on acid-free paper
Version Date: 20160502

International Standard Book Number-13: 978-1-4987-4935-0 (Hardback)

Visit the Taylor & Francis Web site at
http://www.taylorandfrancis.com

and the CRC Press Web site at
http://www.crcpress.com

Contents

5 Regenerative Medicine for Multimodal Management of Osteoarthritis   133

Preface

'Multimodal' has become a popular term in the recent medical literature. Arguably introduced as an acronym for 'balanced anesthesia', denoting induction by a multiple drug approach, multimodal is currently recognized to identify any protocol that includes multiple drugs, agents, adjuncts or delivery methods. Marketers have also come to embrace the term, as they tout the virtues of administering their products as part of a given protocol. Frequently this leads to advertising, where one is encouraged to incorporate a given product within 'your multimodal protocol'. Herein, at issue is actually identifying a foundation protocol.

The **Multimodal Management of Osteoarthritis** described in this work delineates an evidence-based approach for the canine patient with osteoarthritis (OA), pursuing the objective of the best available medicine. Appreciating that surgical intervention may initially be required, particularly for stabilizing a joint, the major focus of this work is the 'conservative' management of OA. A simplistic approach is taken with the overlapping of two three-pointed triangles of management: medical and non-medical. Medical management includes nonsteroidal anti-inflammatory drugs (NSAIDs), chondroprotectant and adjunct agents; while the non-medical management includes weight-control/exercise, an eicosapentaenoic acid-rich diet and physical rehabilitation. Each of these approaches has been independently shown to be effective, and while there are no published works on their collective synergism, the concept is intuitive and three actual case examples are overviewed.

As we learn more about the pathophysiology of OA, we are also becoming more aware of how to implement treatments to attack various components of these pathways. Our challenge as veterinary health professionals is to maintain awareness of contemporary issues in treating OA so that we can offer canine patients the care they need and deserve.

Since publication of this text's first edition (2010), several innovations are now potentially available for consideration in treating the OA patient. First, is introduction of a new Piprant Class, prostaglandin receptor antagonist. This new (2013) class of drugs specifically targets receptor subtypes for prostaglandin E_2; namely EP4, which has been identified as a major player in the pain pathway. This new class of drugs may offer the same analgesic features as NSAIDs, but without the associated adverse effects of many NSAIDs. Second, is availability of a new therapeutic and diagnostic tool to treat canine joint inflammation using radiosynoviorthesis. With the novel preparation of the radionuclide tin-117m suspended in a colloid (homogenous tin-117m colloid), comes a practical and safe treatment option for those patients that either respond poorly or have adverse side effects with traditional therapies. Because this treatment option is quite novel to companion animal practice, a detailed overview is provided in this revised text edition. The author would like to thank Drs. John Donecker and Nigel Stevenson for their inclusive contribution to insights on this treatment. Third, is recognition of the role that stem cells and platelet rich plasma are increasingly playing in the management of OA. The author expresses his deep appreciation for the segment on regenerative medicine provided by Drs. Sherman Canapp and Brittany Jean Carr (Veterinary Orthopedic Sports Medicine Group, Annapolis Junction, MD, USA).

This textbook is intended for veterinary healthcare professionals seeking to better understand the issues related to pain management associated with canine OA.

Disclaimer

Knowledge and information in this field are constantly changing. As new information and experience become available, changes in treatments and therapies may become necessary. The reader is advised to check current information regarding the procedures described in this book, the manufacturer of each product administered to verify the recommended dose or formula, the method and duration of administration, and any contraindications. Where a particular pharmaceutical is not approved for use in the target species and reader's country, the reader accepts full responsibility for administration. It is the responsibility of the reader to make an appropriate diagnosis, determine the dosages and the best treatments for each individual patient, and to take all appropriate safety precautions, including informed consent of the owner. To the fullest extent of the law, neither the Publisher nor the Authors assume any liability for any injury and/or damage to persons or property arising out of, or related to, any use of the material contained in this book.

Abbreviations

AA	arachidonic acid	GaAs	gallium-arsenide
ACE	angiotensin-converting enzyme	GAG	glycosaminoglycan
ADE	adverse drug event	GAIT	Glucosamine/chondroitin Arthritis Intervention Trial
ADPC	adipose derived cultured progenitor cells	GI	gastrointestinal
AL-TENS	acupuncture-like transcutaneous electrical nerve stimulation	GS	glucosamine sulfate
		HA	hyaluronic acid
ALA	alpha-lipoic acid	HFT	high frequency transcutaneous electrical nerve stimulation
ALT	alanine aminotransferase		
AMA	American Medical Association	HRQL	health-related quality of life
ANA	antinuclear antibody	HTC	homogenous tin-117m colloid
ASU	avocado/soybean unsaponifiable	ICAM	intercellular cell adhesion molecule 1
bFGF	basic fibroblast growth factor	IFN	interferon
BAPS	biomechanical ankle platform system	IL	interleukin
BMAC	bone marrow aspirate concentrate	iNOS	inducible nitric oxide synthase
BMSC	bone marrow derived stem cells	IRAP	IL-1 receptor antagonist protein
CAM	complementary and alternative medicine	IVD	intervertebral disc
		keV	kiloelectron volt
CCL	cranial cruciate ligament	LE	lupus erythematosus
CCLT	cranial cruciate ligament transection	LFT	low frequency transcutaneous electrical nerve stimulation
CK	creatine kinase		
CNS	central nervous system	LLLT	low-level laser therapy
CODI	Cincinnati Orthopedic Disability Index	LOX	lipoxygenase
COX	cyclo-oxygenase	LPS	lipopolysaccharide
CT	computed tomography	LR-PRP	leukocyte-rich platelet rich plasma
DHA	docosahexaenoic acid	LP-PRP	leukocyte-poor platelet rich plasma
DJD	degenerative joint disease	MMP	matrix metalloproteinase
DMOAA	disease modifying osteoarthritic agent	MRI	magnetic resonance imaging
DMOAD	disease modifying osteoarthritic drug	MSC	mesenchymal stem cell
ECG	electrocardiography	nAchR	nicotinic acetylcholine receptor
ECGC	epigallocatechin gallate (antioxidant)	NCCAM	U.S. National Center of Complementary and Alternative Medicine
EGF	epidermal growth factor		
EMG	electromyography	NF-κB	nuclear factor kappa-light-chain-enhancer of activated B cells
EPA	eicosapentaenoic acid		
ES	electrical stimulation	NIH	National Institutes of Health
ESWT	extracorporeal shock wave therapy	NMDA	N-methyl-D-aspartate
FCP	fragmented coronoid process	NMES	neuromuscular electrical stimulation
FDA	Food and Drug Administration	NNT	number needed to treat
GABA	γ-aminobutyric acid	NO	nitric oxide
GaAlA	gallium-aluminum-arsenide	NRS	numeric rating scale

NSAID	nonsteroidal anti-inflammatory drug
OA	osteoarthritis
OCD	osteochondritis dissecans
OTC	over-the-counter
PAG	periaqueductal gray
PBS	phosphate-buffered saline
PDGF	platelet-derived growth factor
PENS	percutaneous electrical nerve stimulation
PG	prostaglandin
Piprants	new (Y2013) drug class of prostaglandin E2 receptor antagonists
PKC	protein kinase C
PLA	phospholipase A
POMR	problem oriented medical record
PPI	proton pump inhibitor
PRGF	plasma rich in growth factors
PRP	platelet-rich plasma
PSGAG	polysulfated glycosaminoglycan
QOL	quality of life
RA	rheumatoid arthritis
RBC	red blood cell
RCCT	randomized, controlled, patient-centered clinical trials
RNA	ribonucleic acid
ROM	range of motion
RSO	radiosynoviorthesis
RSV	radiosynovectomy
SAP	serum alkaline phosphatase
SDS	simple descriptive scale
SMF	static magnet fields
SRI	serotonin reuptake inhibitor
SVF	stromal vascular fraction
TCA	tricyclic antidepressant
TCM	traditional Chinese medicine
TENS	transcutaneous electrical nerve stimulation
TGF	transforming growth factor
TIMP	tissue inhibiting metalloproteinase
Tin-117m (Sn-117m)	an artificially produced radionuclide of tin
TNF	tumor necrosis factor
TPI	total pressure index
TX	thromboxane
UAP	ununited anconeal process
US	ultrasound
VAS	visual analog scale
VCAM	vascular cell adhesion molecule
VCPG	viable cells per gram
VEGF	vascular endothelial growth factor
VRS	verbal rating scale

Chapter 1

Pain and Lameness

PAIN

Pain is the clinical sign most frequently associated with osteoarthritis (OA)[1]. The clinical manifestation of this pain is lameness. When an animal presents with clinical lameness, a determination must be made whether the animal is unable to use the limb, or is unwilling to use the limb. Inability to use the limb may be attributable to musculoskeletal changes, such as joint contracture or muscle atrophy. These anomalies are best addressed with physical rehabilitation. On the other hand, unwillingness to use a limb is most often attributable to pain. Herein, lameness is an avoidance behavior.

Ironically, articular cartilage is frequently the focus of studies regarding OA. However, clinical treatment of the OA patient is most often focused on the alleviation of pain. Appreciating that articular cartilage is aneural, the focus of OA pain management resides in the periarticular structures. No pain is elicited by stimulation of cartilage, and stimulation of normal synovial tissue rarely evokes pain[2].

OA pain is the result of a complex interplay between structural change, biochemical alterations, peripheral and central pain-processing mechanisms, and individual cognitive processing of nociception (**1.1**).

The source of pain in the joint 'organ' is multifocal: direct stimulation of the joint capsule and bone receptors by cytokines/ligands of inflammatory and degradative processes, physical stimulation of the joint capsule from distension (effusion) and stretch (laxity, subluxation, abnormal articulation), physical stimulation of subchondral bone from abnormal loading, and (likely) physical stimulation of muscle, tendon, and ligaments.

Bony changes at the joint margins and beneath areas of damaged cartilage can be major sources of OA pain. Subchondral bone contains unmyelinated nerve fibers, which increase in number with OA[3]. Increased pressure on subchondral bone (associated with OA) results in stimulation of these nociceptors. This is thought to contribute to the vague, but consistent pain frequently associated with OA. In humans OA is believed to be responsible for increased intraosseous pressure, which may contribute to chronic pain, particularly nocturnal pain. Human OA patients report pain, even at rest, associated with raised intraosseous pressure[4].

LAMENESS

Most often lameness in pets is identified by the owner, who subsequently seeks further consultation and advice from their veterinarian, or is identified by the veterinarian during routine examination. Most simply, dogs (and cats) are lame because they cannot or will not use one or more limbs in a normal fashion. Pain associated with OA is recognized to become more persistent and intense as the disease progresses. The condition may be asymptomatic in the early stages. With progression of the disease, discomfort may be continuous, or exacerbated by motion and weight bearing. In the later stages of OA, pain can become pervasive and affect nearly all activities and behaviors.

DIAGNOSIS OF OA

A proper diagnosis depends on a complete history and full assessment of the patient, possibly including:
- A complete physical, orthopedic, and neurologic examination.
- Radiographs of affected area(s).
- Advanced imaging, such as computed tomography, magnetic resonance imaging, nuclear scintigraphy.

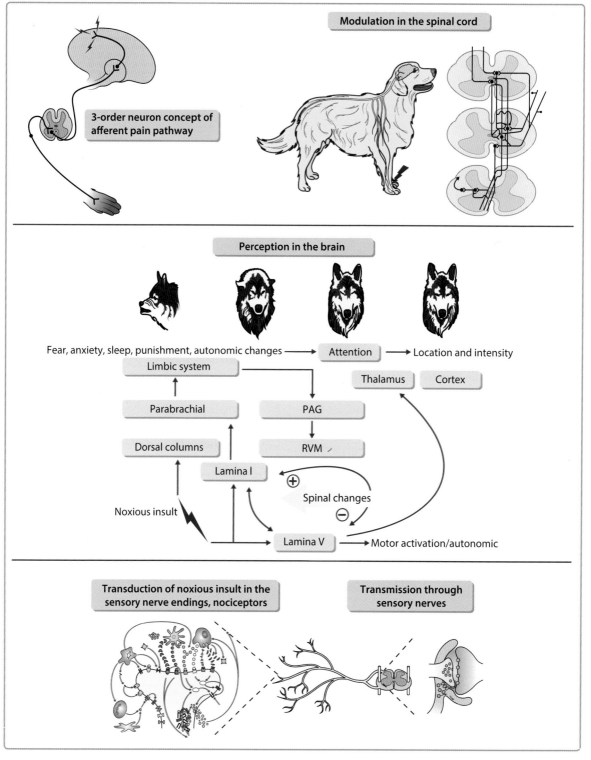

1.1 The pain associated with osteoarthritis is far more complex than the 3-order neuron 'pathway'. Many sophisticated processes occur in the functions of transduction, transmission, modulation, and perception. PAG: periaqueductal grey; RVM: rostral ventromedial medulla.

- Advanced gait analysis, such as force plate (kinetic) analysis of gait and motion (kinematic) analysis.
- Clinicopathologic examination including hematology and serum chemistries, especially creatine kinase and electrolytes, and synovial fluid analysis.
- Electrodiagnostic testing: ultrasound, electromyography, nerve conduction velocity measurements, evoked potential recordings with repetitive nerve stimulation.
- Muscle biopsy examination including histopathology and histochemical analysis.
- Special tests: muscle percussion, serology for pathogens (e.g. *Neospora*, *Toxoplasma*), measurement of acetylcholine receptor antibody, immunohistochemistry, and molecular diagnostic techniques.

ANAMNESIS

The medical history, signalment, and owner's complaint(s) comprise the process of anamnesis. Most canine patients do not vocalize from their pain of OA, and many pet owners do not believe their pet is in pain if it does not vocalize. Nevertheless, signs suggesting animal discomfort include lameness, muscle atrophy, reluctance to exercise, general malaise, lethargy, inappetence or anorexia, change in temperament, licking or biting an affected joint, restlessness, insomnia, seeking warmth, seeking comfortable bedding, and difficulty posturing to toilet. Supraspinal influences are known to alter the behavior of humans with OA[1], and it is reasonable to presume the same occurs in dogs.

Pet owners often recognize lameness only when there is gait asymmetry; however, dogs with bilateral OA, such as with hip or elbow dysplasia, have a symmetrically abnormal gait and do not favor a single limb. These patients shift weight from hind to forelimbs or vice versa with resultant muscle atrophy of the affected limbs and increased development in compensating limbs. Rarely are dogs nonweight bearing simply due to OA. Pet owners do often report that their dog is stiff after resting, particularly following strenuous exercise, but they report that the pet will 'warm out of the stiffness'.

The amount of time required to warm out of this stiffness gradually increases with progression of the disease. Pet owners also frequently report a shortened stride and stiff gait. This is associated with a decreased range of motion (ROM) in the joint, often due to joint capsule fibrosis and osteophyte formation.

EXAMINATION

For many years degenerative joint disease (DJD) (often used interchangeably with the term OA) was considered a disease of the cartilage. DJD is most appropriately considered a disease of the entire joint, with the influence of multiple structures including articular cartilage. Pain is a hallmark of DJD, provoked by instability, and therefore a comprehensive physical examination is the essential diagnostic tool.

An orthopedic examination should be part of every routine examination and should be conducted in conjunction with a neurologic examination (when appropriate) to identify neurologic causes for pain or lameness, such as a nerve root signature sign secondary to a laterally herniated intervertebral disc (IVD) or brachial plexus pathology.

A consistent 'routine' for examining a patient is advised, and it is also recommended that the 'lame' limb be examined last. A consistent examination pattern (e.g. distal limb to proximal limb, and left side to right side or vice versa) is helpful to avoid missing a structure during the examination, and leaving the most painful limb for last in the examination avoids the early elicitation of pain which may render the patient noncompliant for further examination. A thorough examination also requires the aid of an assistant who is adequately trained to hold and restrain the animal. The assistant is also important for identifying the animal's painful response to examination, such as body shifts and change of facial expression.

Animal restraint
Appropriate animal restraint by the assistant (with the patient standing on the examination table) is with one arm over or under the patient's trunk, while the other arm is placed under and around

the patient's neck (**1.2A**). This constraint allows the assistant to quickly tighten his/her grip to control the animal and avoid the patient from harming anyone, should it become confrontational. In lateral recumbency the assistant should be at the animal's dorsum, 'lightly leaning' on the animal with his/her forearms while holding the hind and forelimbs (**1.2B**). One forearm should be placed on the animal's neck, with that hand grasping the forelimb that is closest to the table, or the 'down limb'. The other arm is placed over the top of the abdomen and the hand grasps the 'down' hindlimb. With this restraint, the assistant can rapidly increase his/her amount of weight on their forearms, thereby controlling the animal's movements. Regarding restraint, large dogs are analogous to horses: if you control their head, you control their body.

THE ORTHOPEDIC EXAMINATION

Forelimb examination

In the growing dog, forelimb lameness differentials mostly reflect abnormal stressors on normal bone or normal stressors on abnormal bone (excluding fractures and minor soft tissue injuries) and include:
- Osteochondritis dissecans (OCD): shoulder.
- Luxation/subluxation shoulder: congenital.
- Avulsion: supraglenoid tubercle.
- OCD: elbow.
- Ununited anconeal process (UAP).
- Fragmented coronoid process (FCP).
- Ununited medial epicondyle.
- Elbow incongruity:
  - congenital.
  - physical injury.
- Premature closure of growth plates, such as with radius curvus.
- Retained cartilaginous core (ulna).
- Panosteitis* (a disease of diaphyseal bone).
- Hypertrophic osteodystrophy*.

In the adult dog, forelimb lameness differentials mostly reflect abnormal stressors on normal bone or normal stressors on abnormal bone (excluding fractures and minor soft tissue injuries) and include:
- Arthritis.
- OCD: shoulder.
- Luxation /subluxation: shoulder.

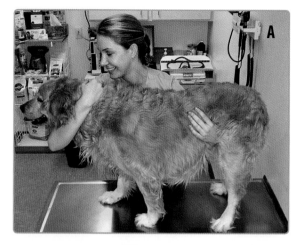

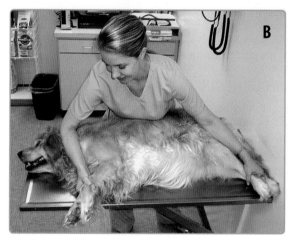

1.2 Restraint for examination. Standing restraint (**A**) of large dogs is done with the neck cradled close to the assistant's chest with one arm, while the other arm controls the patient's trunk by placement either under or over the trunk. If the patient struggles or becomes aggressive, the assistant holds the dog as tight as possible. Lateral restraint (**B**) of large dogs is done with the assistant's forearm over the dog's neck. If the patient struggles, more weight is applied on the forearm.

- Avulsion: supraglenoid tubercle.
- Bicipital tenosynovitis*.
- Calcification of supraspinatus tendon*.
- Contracture of infra- or supraspinatus*.
- Medial glenohumeral laxity.
- OCD: elbow.
- UAP.

- FCP.
- Ununited medial epicondyle.
- Elbow incongruity.
- Angular limb deformity.
- Hypertrophic osteopathy.
- Bone/soft tissue neoplasia*.
- Inflammatory arthritis.

* denote pathology/disease conditions which are not considered OA, but often manifest similar clinical presentations.

For the purpose of examination, the forelimb can be anatomically segmented into the paw, antebrachium, brachium, scapula, and interpositional joints. Although the entire limb should be examined in every patient, the orthopedic examination can be focused more on areas prone to disease and signalment of the individual patient.

Paw

The paw should be thoroughly examined with flexion and extension of each digit, as well as inspection of each nail and nail bed. Findings incidental to those suggesting OA might include:

- Pad lacerations.
- Foreign bodies.
- Split nails.
- Overgrown nails.
- Nail bed tumors.
- Phalangeal luxations/fractures.

Some patients resist manipulation of the paws. Here, the assistant can be very helpful by talking to the patient or scratching the patient to distract him/her from the examination.

Carpus

The carpus should be placed under stress in flexion, extension, valgus, and varus (**1.3–1.6**). The normal

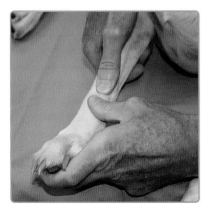

1.3 Carpus flexion. The carpus should be comfortably flexed with the palmar surface nearly touching the flexor surface of the antebrachium.

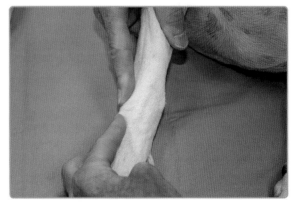

1.5 Placing the carpus in valgus stress identifies integrity of the medial radial collateral ligament.

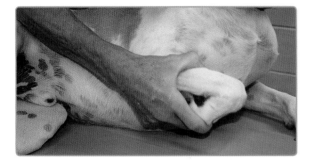

1.4 The carpus should be stressed in extension, looking for signs of discomfort/ pain.

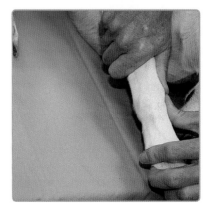

1.6 Placing a varus stress on the carpus challenges the integrity of the lateral ulnar collateral ligament.

carpus should flex comfortably until the palmar surface of the paw nearly touches the flexor surface of the antebrachium. Findings from the carpal examination may include:

- Young dog 'carpal laxity syndrome'.
- Carpal flexural deformity of young dogs.
- Degenerative joint disease.
- Hyperextension.
- Inflammatory arthritis.
- Luxation.
- Fracture (including an intra-articular fracture, possibly mistaken as OA).

Joint capsule distension is easily palpated and suggests joint inflammation.

Antebrachium

Periosteum of bone is a sensitive tissue, well innervated with nociceptive axons. Therefore, examination of both the radius and ulna should focus on deep palpation for a response of bone pain (**1.7**). Panosteitis is commonly revealed in this manner. Osteosarcoma is another condition that results in pain on palpation of the metaphyseal region of bones. Although an orthopedic examination would include assessment of the antebrachium, OA includes only diarthrodial joints. Nevertheless, joint pain should be localized and differentiated from the pain of long bones and soft tissues.

Physeal disturbances are relatively common in the growing dog, the severity of which depends on the amount of growth remaining following injury until physeal closure. Resultant aberrant growth is expressed as angular limb deformities of the carpus and/or the elbow. In general, the plane of the elbow joint should be parallel to the plane of the carpal joint.

Sources of lameness within the radius/ulna include:

- Hypertrophic osteopathy.
- Angular limb deformities.
- Panosteitis.
- Neoplasia.
- Hypertrophic osteodystrophy.

Elbow

The elbow is the most common forelimb joint responsible for lameness, especially in growing dogs of predisposed breeds (i.e. large breeds, sporting dogs, and Rottweilers). The elbow should be

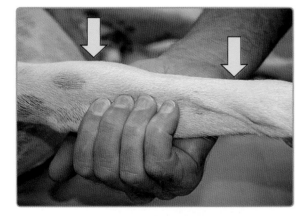

1.7 Digital palpation is made on the antero-medial aspect of the antebrachium, where there is minimal muscle cover. In the normal dog the elbow joint is parallel to the carpal joint.

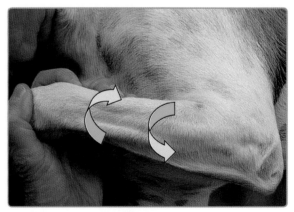

1.8 Examination of the elbow joint includes manipulation through a full range of motion.

manipulated through a complete ROM (**1.8**), noting the abnormal presence of crepitus or painful response, particularly in full extension. In a normal dog, hyperextension of the elbow should elicit minimal to no discomfort. Valgus and varus stress placed upon the joint are performed to assess integrity of the joint capsule and collateral ligaments/tendons. Joint effusion accompanying disease often distends the joint, palpable by placement of the thumb and index finger in the normally concave depression caudal to the distal humeral epicondyles.

Common orthopedic diseases of the elbow joint include FCP, UAP, and OCD. Palpation of the medial joint, in the area of the medial coronoid, often elicits a painful response in dogs suffering from any (or all) of these conditions (**1.9, 1.10**).

Less common findings of the elbow, aside from OA, include:

- Subluxations or luxation (can be associated with OA).
- Fractures.
- Radioulnar incongruities (can be associated with OA).
- Inflammatory arthropathies.
- Neoplasia.

Brachium

Osteosarcoma is a common tumor of the forelimb, frequently residing in the proximal humerus (and distal radius/ulna). Deep palpation along the length of the humerus is conducted to reveal evidence of pain and areas of inflammation or swelling. Other abnormal conditions of the brachium (not associated with OA) include:

- Hypertrophic osteodystrophy.
- Fractures.
- Hypertrophic osteopathy.
- Panosteitis.

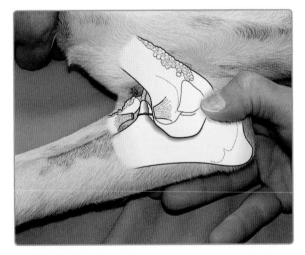

1.9 Fragmented medial coronoid, ununited anconeal process, and osteochondritis are common diseases of the elbow, constituting elbow dysplasia. Patients with any of these pathologies often resent deep digital pressure on the medial aspect of the joint near the affected location. Further, joint capsule distension is common with any of these conditions, and can best be identified with palpation, as with thumb placement in the figure.

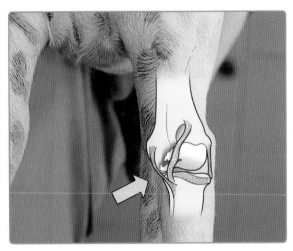

1.10 Osteochondritis dissecans of the elbow most commonly occurs on the distal, medial humeral condyle.

Shoulder

As with examination of all joints, the shoulder joint should be examined through a full ROM to include flexion, extension, adduction, and abduction as well as internal and external rotation (**1.11**). Of particular note is examination of the shoulder joint in extension. The examiner should be mindful to avoid placing the forelimb into extension with his/her hand placed caudal or distal to the elbow joint (**1.12**). Placing the hand behind or distal to the elbow when forcing the shoulder into extension also forces the elbow into extension. A resultant painful response from the patient might actually be from elbow disease rather than shoulder disease. The examiner's hand placed above the elbow allows the elbow to be placed in a neutral position, and avoids this complication.

Painful conditions associated with the shoulder joint include:

- OCD (especially in young animals, which can lead to OA).
- Biceps tenosynovitis.
- Mineralization of the supraspinatus.
- Infraspinatus contracture.
- DJD (of unknown etiology).
- Articular fractures.
- Incomplete ossification of the caudal glenoid process.
- Medial shoulder instability (leading to OA).

- Luxation, either congenital or acquired (leading to OA).

Stabilization of the shoulder joint is maintained by both medial and lateral glenohumeral ligaments, the shape of the articular surfaces (humeral head and glenoid), and musculotendinous units of the rotator cuff: the supraspinatus, infraspinatus, teres minor, and subscapularis. Abnormal excursion of the shoulder joint, with or without pain, suggests involvement of several of these periarticular soft tissue structures. Medial shoulder instability

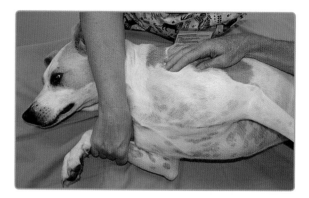

1.11 Examination of the shoulder in flexion. The shoulder joint should also be assessed in abduction and adduction. Note restraint of the patient with the assistant's forearm over the patient's neck.

1.12 Avoid placing the forelimb in extension with hand placement caudal to the elbow. This typically causes simultaneous hyperextension of the elbow and may give a false impression that the source of discomfort is in the shoulder joint when it may reside in the elbow joint.

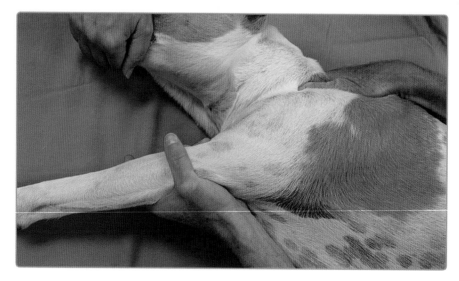

typically results in excessive shoulder abduction as well as pain at the end of abduction.

Scapula

The scapula is not a common source of forelimb pain. However, atrophy of scapular muscles is frequently associated with disuse of the forelimb as well as many neurologic conditions. Tumors, acromion fractures, midbody fractures, and scapular luxation from the thoracic wall are commonly seen when pain is localized to the scapular area, so deep palpation and manipulation of the scapula should be performed when this anatomic structure is suspect.

The biceps tendon should be palpated from its origin on the supraglenoid tubercle through its excursion within the intertubercular groove in the proximal humerus. Biceps tenosynovitis frequently results in the patient's painful response to this deep palpation (1.13). Another maneuver that may elicit pain is to flex the shoulder joint while simultaneously extending the elbow joint. This places maximal stretch on the biceps tendon and may exacerbate a pain response.

Spine

IVD disease and lumbosacral disease commonly lead to limb dysfunction. Therefore, examination of the patient's spine should be part of an orthopedic/neurologic examination (1.14). Deep palpation of the paravertebral musculature with the patient in extension of the spine often reveals peripheral neuropathies and spinal pathology. DJD of the spinal articular facets is not uncommon in IVD disease and instability. Further, clinical presentation of caudal spinal disease can mimic the pain associated with hip dysplasia.

Hindlimb examination

In the growing dog, hindlimb lameness differentials mostly reflect abnormal stressors on normal bone or normal stressors on abnormal bone (excluding fractures and minor soft tissue injuries) and include:
- Hip dysplasia.
- Avascular necrosis: femoral head (Legg–Calvé–Perthes)*.
- OCD: stifle.
- Luxating patella complex.

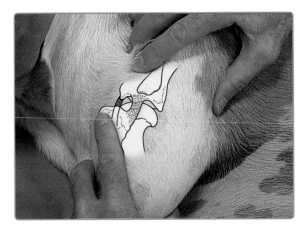

1.13 Examination of the shoulder joint with superimposed arthrology. A 'drawer manipulation' of the shoulder joint should be part of the examination, as well as palpation of the biceps tendon (red) from its origin on the supraglenoid tubercle of the scapula through the intertubercular groove of the humerus.

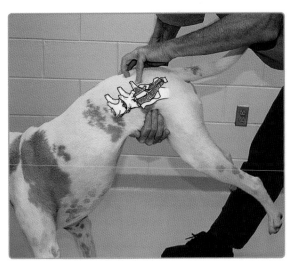

1.14 Lumbosacral (or intervertebral disc) disease can often manifest as hip or limb disease, therefore palpation of the spine should be included as part of an orthopedic examination.

- Genu valgum (knock knee).
- OCD: hock.
- Avulsion of long digital extensor*.
- Panosteitis*.
- Hypertrophic osteodystrophy*.

*   denote pathology/disease conditions which are not considered OA, but often manifest similar clinical presentations.

Adult dog hindlimb lameness differentials mostly reflect abnormal stressors on normal bone or normal stressors on abnormal bone (excluding fractures and minor soft tissue injuries) and include:
- Arthritis.
- Hip dysplasia.
- OCD: stifle.
- Cruciate/meniscal syndrome.
- Luxating patella complex.
- Genu valgum.
- Avulsion of long digital extensor*.
- Luxation of superficial digital flexor tendon*.
- Inflammatory arthritis.
- Neoplasia*.

*   denote pathology/disease conditions which are not considered OA, but often manifest similar clinical presentations.

As with the forelimb, the hindlimb can be divided into anatomic regions: paw, tarsus, tibia/fibula, stifle or knee, femur, hip, and pelvis. Cranial cruciate ligament compromise of the stifle and hip dysplasia constitute two of the most common DJD conditions causing pain/lameness in the dog.

Paw

Examination of the hind paws is similar to examination of the fore paws. Each individual digit, including the nail and nail bed, should be assessed.

Tarsus

The tarsocrural joint accounts for ROM in flexion and extension (**1.15, 1.16**). Popping of the joint, palpated during ROM assessment, may be associated with displacement of the superficial digital flexor tendon following retinaculum tearing. This condition can lead to hyperflexion of the tarsus and

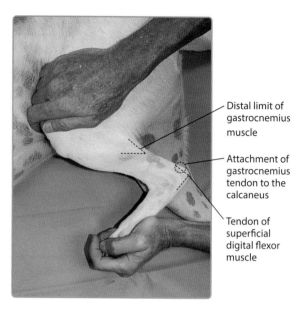

Distal limit of gastrocnemius muscle

Attachment of gastrocnemius tendon to the calcaneus

Tendon of superficial digital flexor muscle

1.15 Examination of the tibiotarsal (hock) joint in flexion. Compromise of the gastrocnemius tendon and superficial digital flexor muscle tendon is best identified with this joint in flexion.

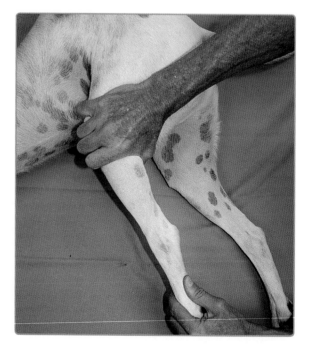

1.16 Examination of the tibiotarsal joint in extension. Examination of this joint should include palpation of the joint capsule, looking for distension.

digits. Damage to the common calcaneal tendon can also lead to tarsal hyperflexion. Assessing this tendon from its insertion on the calcaneus, proximally to the gastrocnemius muscles should be performed with a clinical presentation of hyperflexion.

The tarsocrural joint can also show instability resulting from trauma. Placing the joint in both varus and valgus stress evaluates the collateral ligaments that maintain the structural integrity of this hinge joint. The tarsocrural joint is also predisposed in some breeds to OCD (both the medial and lateral ridges of the talus). OCD is often accompanied by distension of the joint capsule, palpable on the dorsal as well as the caudomedial and caudolateral joint surfaces.

Tibia and fibula

The medial aspect of the tibia has little soft tissue cover, making the identification of osseous abnormalities relatively easy during palpation. Deep palpation is required on the lateral aspect of the tibia and fibula, where there is considerable proximal muscle mass. Lameness and pain of the tibia and fibula (not considered OA) can arise from:

- Panosteitis.
- Hypertrophic osteodystrophy.
- Physeal fractures (possibly with associated limb deformity).
- Physeal disturbances.
- Neoplasia.
- Limb deformity (often associated with patellar luxation) (which can contribute to OA).
- Fractures.

Stifle

Examination of the stifle is most informative when performed in both the standing and laterally recumbent positions. Both stifles are examined simultaneously by approaching the standing patient caudally and wrapping your fingers from lateral to medial around the patellae. This allows comparison of one limb with the other and easier determination of the presence of a 'medial buttress' – a firm swelling medial to the joint, often associated with long-standing cruciate disease. In this same position of examination, both patellae can be manipulated, assessing for luxation. An attempt should be made to luxate each patella through a range of stifle flexion and extension (**1.17**). Most luxating patellae are apparent in extension. Surprisingly, the most severe patellar luxations can be the most difficult to detect, because severe (grade IV) luxations are commonly

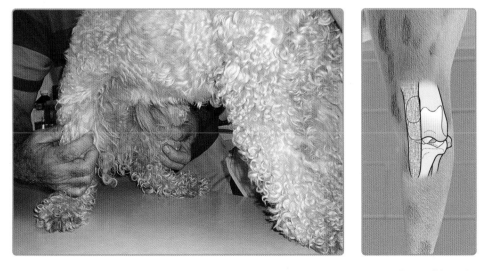

1.17 Bilateral patella assessment should be conducted on each patient, especially small breed dogs. In the more pronounced presentation of medial luxated patella (grade IV) the patella permanently resides medial to the distal, medial trochlear ridge of the femur. This is often accompanied by a medial rotation of the tibia.

associated with fibrosis of the patella outside the trochlear groove, giving the false impression that the patella is properly seated because it cannot be displaced. In these cases, the patella may be located by finding the tibial tuberosity, and palpating proximally along the patellar ligament until the patella is located. The trochlear groove (if one is present in such cases) may be palpated in the central region of the distal femur and compared with the position of the patella to confirm that it is ectopic.

Osteosarcoma is a common tumor type found in the hindlimb, most frequently in the distal femur or proximal tibia. Stretching of the periosteum by expansile tumors sensitizes the periosteum to a painful response with deep palpation.

Examination of the stifle in lateral recumbency begins with assessment of ROM, noting the patient's response to pain. Clicking or popping during this manipulation may indicate meniscal pathology. Assessment of cruciate ligament integrity is made by the cranial tibial thrust maneuver and/or a cranial drawer test (**1.18–1.20**).

Disease conditions of the stifle include:
- Cruciate ligament disease.
- Meniscal disease.
- Patellar luxation.
- OCD.
- Collateral ligament injury.
- Stifle luxation.
- Long digital extensor tendon injury (not associated with OA).

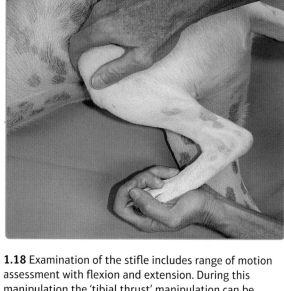

1.18 Examination of the stifle includes range of motion assessment with flexion and extension. During this manipulation the 'tibial thrust' manipulation can be performed to further examine the cranial cruciate ligament. For this test, the index finger of one hand is extended from the patella along the patella tendon to the tibial crest. With the other hand, the hock is flexed until tension of the common calcanean tendon is achieved. If the cranial cruciate ligament is ruptured, the tensed gastrocnemius muscle pushes the tibia forward in relation to the femur, which is palpable by movement of the index finger along the patella tendon.

1.19 Anterior cruciate ligament rupture is a common injury to the stifle. Several specific diagnostics help to identify this condition: the 'tibial thrust' manipulation, a firm swelling in the region of the medial collateral stifle ligament termed 'medial buttress', and the 'drawer' test.

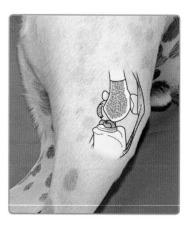

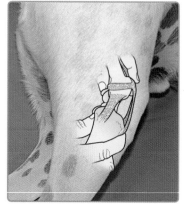

1.20 The 'drawer' test is used to determine cruciate ligament stability. The thumb of one hand is placed on the lateral fabella and the index finger over the patella. The thumb of the other hand is placed on the fibular head with the index finger placed on the tibial crest. An attempt is then made to move the tibia cranially (positive cranial drawer) or caudally (positive caudal drawer) relative to the femur.

Femur

Palpation along the length of the femur should be performed, searching for swelling and pain. Pathologic conditions of the femur not associated with OA may include:

- Hypertrophic osteopathy.
- Hypertrophic osteodystrophy.
- Panosteitis.
- Neoplasia.
- Fracture.
- Limb deformity (often associated with patella luxation).

Hip

The hip is a common source of pain, especially in older dogs. Hip dysplasia is a common orthopedic disease, particularly in large breeds, and tends to manifest with pain in a biphasic pattern, occurring near skeletal maturity and when the animal enters its 'senior years' (**1.21–1.23**). The most revealing examination technique for hip dysplasia in young dogs is the Ortolani examination, which tests for laxity of the coxofemoral joint. This is best performed under sedation or general anesthesia with the patient in lateral or dorsal recumbency. The femur is forced in a dorsal, axial direction with one hand on the flexed stifle and the other hand over the hip/pelvis. In the presence of hip laxity, the hand over the pelvis will detect subluxation when the femoral head moves dorsally and laterally 'up and over' the acetabular rim. Maintaining the axial force, the femur is then slowly abducted, allowing the femoral head to once again reduce into the acetabulum. A palpable (and occasionally audible)

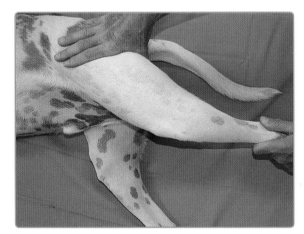

1.21 Examination of the hip joint in extension.

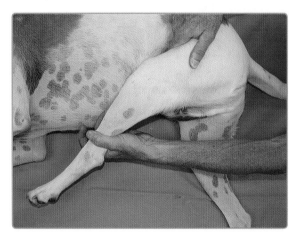

1.22 Examination of the hip joint in flexion.

1.23 Ventrodorsal radiographic positioning for assessment of hip dysplasia. The overlay demonstrates subluxation of the coxofemoral joint.

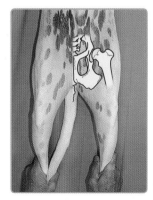

'clunk' is detected in the 'positive Ortolani maneuver', confirming coxofemoral laxity (**1.24**). Digital rectal palpation might be further informative in animals showing signs of pelvic pain.

Other orthopedic conditions of the hip, exclusive of OA, include:

- Neoplasia.
- Fractures.
- Inflammatory arthropathies.
- Physeal fractures (e.g. capital physis in skeletally immature dogs).

Table 1.1 presents the normal ROM for canine joints.

DIAGNOSTIC IMAGING

The foundation for diagnosing OA is the physical examination. Diagnostic imaging is a logical next step in a diagnostic sequence. The indications for diagnostic imaging include: to confirm or refute a clinically suspected lesion, to suggest or document the site of a suspected lesion, to characterize the nature and extent of a known or suspected lesion, to follow the progression of disease or healing, to aid in establishing prognosis, to plan or evaluate

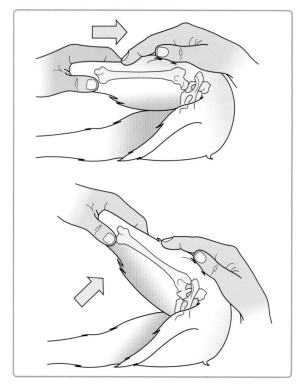

1.24 A positive Ortolani sign is the most revealing diagnostic manipulation for hip dysplasia.

Table 1.1 Normal range of motion for canine joints

Joint	Range of motion*	
Shoulder (relative to the spine of the scapula)	Flexion to 57°	
		Extension to 165°
Elbow (relative to the axis of the humerus)	Flexion to 36°	
		Extension to 166°
Carpus (relative to the antebrachium)	Flexion to 32°	
		Extension to 196°
Hip (relative to the axis of the pelvis)	Flexion to 50°	
		Extension to 162°
Stifle (relative to the femur)	Flexion to 41°	
		Extension to 162°
Tarsus (relative to the tibia with the stifle at 90°)	Flexion to 38°	
		Extension to 165°

*These data should be used as a guide, interpreted together with the clinician's experience and comparison with the contralateral joint. (Data from: Reliability of goniometry in Labrador retrievers. Jaegger G, Marcellin-Little DJ, Levine D. *Am J Vet Res* 2002;**63**:979–86.)

surgical therapies, to suggest or guide additional diagnostic procedures, and to screen for diseases with obscure clinical signs[5].

Survey radiography

Evaluation on conventional radiographs of the osteoarthritic joint should include: narrowing or ablation of the joint space with radiographs taken in standing position, increased density to the sub-chondral bone (eburnation), new bone formation of joint margins (osteophytosis), joint deformity with preservation of articular margins, proliferative and lytic changes at the attachment sites of the joint capsule and supporting ligaments, meniscal calcifi-cation, and partial-to-complete ankylosis. Amongst these, osteophytosis, subchondral bone sclerosis, remodeling, and joint space narrowing are the most common.

Osteophytes are characteristic of OA, develop in areas of the joint subject to low stress, and are usually marginal (peripheral). The osteophyte is believed to form from metaplasia of synovium into cartilage with the formation of chondroblasts and cartilage at the margin of the articular surface[6]. Radiographically, osteophytes appear as lips of new bone around the edges of the joint. They develop initially in the periarticular regions covered by the synovial membrane. Periosteal and synovial osteophytes may develop from the periosteum or synovial membrane and are termed buttressing, especially when located at the medial aspect of the stifle joint. Osteophyte formation can develop at the site of bony attachment of the joint capsule or adjacent ligament or tendon insertion, termed enthesophytes. Clinically, osteophytes of the (human) knee are associated with pain and predict pain more accurately than the narrowing of knee joint space in all radiological views[7].

Joint space narrowing, which is considered more accurate on weight-bearing radiographs, has been an accepted indicator of articular cartilage degeneration in human patients[8], although others question its diagnostic value compared to other indirect indicators[9]. The impracticality of obtain-ing weight-bearing radiographs has limited their use for evaluating the joint space in dogs. Areas of the joint that are subject to increased load bearing show subchondral bone changes that accompany OA including eburnation, cyst formation, flatten-ing, and deformity[10].

After localization of the lameness by means of a physical examination, survey radiographs can provide morphologic information about the area of interest. Additional diagnostic imaging can be per-formed based upon the type of information sought and the anatomic structure to be evaluated.

Supplemental diagnostic imaging

Table 1.2 presents a comparison of various imaging modalities in the clinical setting.

ARTHROSCOPY

A variety of joint disorders lend themselves well to the minimally invasive diagnostic and thera-peutic technique of arthroscopy (*Table 1.3*). Lesions are often diagnosed before degenerative changes are radiographically apparent. This is due to the magnification of joint surfaces, joint capsule, and intra-articular structures. Arthroscopy has been used in a variety of situations including: diagnostic evaluation of joints, removal of loose fragments or foreign bodies, debridement with septic arthritis, osteophyte excision, synovectomy with rheuma-toid arthritis (RA), and arthrolysis of contractures. There are few complications associated with arthroscopy, although equipment is expensive and technical expertise is essential. Iatrogenic articular cartilage trauma is often a reflection of the arthros-copist's experience and instrument damage is costly. Knowledge of regional anatomy is essential to the arthroscopist. Swelling following arthroscopy is normally absorbed within 24–48 hours after the procedure, and patient recovery time is frequently reduced compared with arthrotomy.

ARTHROCENTESIS

Further diagnostic testing and treatment can be guided by synovial fluid analysis. Differentiating inflammatory from noninflammatory disease is the first interpretative step with a joint tap. If the condition is then diagnosed as inflammatory, it must be determined whether the process is septic or not. Cytologic examination (number, type, and integrity of the nucleated cells) should be made

Table 1.2 Comparison of imaging modalities

Modality	Advantages/disadvantages
Conventional radiography	* Can lead to definitive or differential diagnosis. * Can define the nature and extent of involvement and characterize aggressiveness of the lesion. * Greater spatial resolution than either MRI or CT. * Two-dimensional display of three-dimensional object gives superimposition of structures that may obscure important features.
Ultrasonography	* Real-time noninvasive evaluation of muscular and tendinous structures. * Does not use ionizing radiation. * Can directly image cartilage (user dependent) and synovium, evaluate amount and nature of joint fluid, and localize periarticular mineralization. * Particularly well suited to evaluation of soft tissue structures. * Limited access to joint regions.
Nuclear medicine (scintigraphy)	* High sensitivity for detecting early disease, as well as disease progression. * Surveys all joints during a single examination. * Lacks spatial resolution. * Involves injection of radiolabeled phosphate compound (e.g. technetium-99m-labeled methylene diphosphonate [^{99m}Tc-MDP]). * Nonspecific. * Expensive, specialty training, special equipment, special licensing.
Computed tomography (CT)	* Whereas conventional radiographs have five radiographic opacities (metal, bone, soft tissues, fat, and air) CT systems can record thousands of separate opacities. * Information is captured by several radiation sensors, converted into a digital file, and viewed as a tomographic slice on a computer screen. * High contrast and resolution of osseous tissues are hallmarks. * CT imparts a perception of depth. * Various image display formats can enhance soft tissue or osseous structures individually. * 'Reconstruction' slices can present data in a plane other than that in which the information was obtained. * Anesthesia or profound sedation is required.
Magnetic resonance imaging (MRI)	* Does not use ionizing radiation. * Excellent tissue contrast. * Can generate images in any plane. * Patient must be motionless (general anesthesia). * Excellent for imaging cruciate ligament damage, elbow dysplasia, IVD, and early detection of articular cartilage destruction. * Costly, requires skilled technical support.

Table 1.3 Applications of arthroscopy

Recommended as follow-up to physical/radiographic signs of:	Arthroscopic diagnoses include:	Arthroscopic therapeutic interventions include:
Joint capsular thickening Increased synovial fluid volume Periarticular swelling	OCD Meniscal injuries Fragmented medial coronoid process	OCD of shoulder, elbow, stifle, and hock Fragmented medial coronoid process Ruptured cranial cruciate ligament
Osteophyte formation Bony sclerosis Narrowed joint space Cartilaginous or osseous defects or deformities Bone chips or fragments Joint laxity	DJD Intra-articular fractures Synovitis Bicipital tendonitis Bicipital tendon rupture Neoplasia	

of all aspirates. Culture and susceptibility testing are recommended in any case of inflammatory arthritis. The cause of nonseptic inflammatory joint disease can be difficult to ascertain, often requiring further diagnostic testing (i.e. rickettsial serology, antinuclear antibody, lupus erythematosus [LE] preparation, rheumatoid factor testing, and so on).

Patients should be adequately restrained for arthrocentesis, often requiring sedation, but rarely general anesthesia. The procedure should be performed aseptically and is well described[11]. In polyarthropathies more than one joint should be sampled, including joints that appear normal (**1.25A–E**).

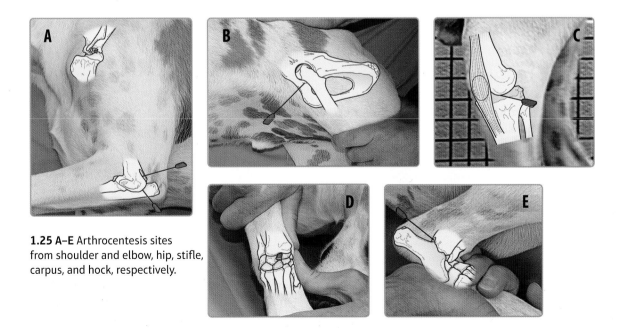

1.25 A–E Arthrocentesis sites from shoulder and elbow, hip, stifle, carpus, and hock, respectively.

QUICK TIPS

Problem oriented medical record

The problem oriented medical record (POMR) is designed for a logical approach to problem solving. Additionally, to avoid overlooking possible differential diagnoses, many find it helpful to screen for disease processes using the DAMNIT acronym of pathophysiology:

- D Degenerative disorders.
- A Anomalies, autoimmunity.
- M Metabolic disorders.
- N Neoplasia, nutritional disorders.
- I Inflammation (infectious or noninfectious), immune disorders, iatrogenic disorders, idiopathic.
- T Toxicity (endogenous or exogenous), trauma (internal or external).

Musculoskeletal disorders:

- Developmental degenerative disorders: agenesis, luxation, ectrodactyly, osteochondrodysplasia, elbow dysplasia (UAP, FCP), growth arrests, growth plate disorders, retained cartilage core; DJD, canine hip dysplasia, cruciate ligament rupture, IVD, lumbosacral instability.
- Autoimmunity: RA, systemic LE.
- Metabolic disorders: panosteitis, osteochondrosis, craniomandibular osteopathy, hypertrophic osteodystrophy, hyperparathyroidism, hyperadrenocorticism.
- Neoplasia: osteosarcoma, chondrosarcoma, hemangiosarcoma, fibrosarcoma, synovial cell sarcoma.
- Nutritional disorders: nutritional secondary hyperparathyroidism, hypervitaminosis A, hypovitaminosis D.
- Inflammation: osteomyelitis, discospondylitis, arthritis.
- Immune-mediated disorders: polyarthritis secondary to trimethoprim sulfa administration.
- Iatrogenic disorders: synostosis.
- Idiopathic: avascular necrosis of the femoral head (Legg–Calvé–Perthes), hypertrophic osteopathy, bone cyst, multiple cartilaginous exostoses.
- Toxicity: lead poisoning.
- Trauma: fracture, luxation, cruciate ligament rupture.

Disease conditions vs. time

Severity of clinical signs can be helpful in differentiating trauma, autoimmune disease, and neoplasia. In trauma, the severity of clinical signs tends to be more acute, while those associated with immune-mediated disease and neoplasia are more chronic or delayed (**1.26**).

Bone disease location vs. disease etiology

Location of the primary disease condition in a bone can often provide insight as to the etiology (**1.27**).

Characteristics and diagnosis of osteoarthritis

Figure **1.28** shows the location of DJD characteristic changes. The diagnosis of OA is made using the methods presented in *Table 1.4*.

Degenerative joint disease:

- Characterized by pain and lameness.
- Diagnosis:
  - physical and orthopedic examination.
  - radiographs.
  - arthroscopy.
  - diagnostic aids.

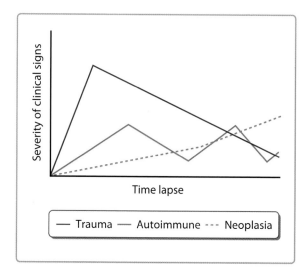

1.26 Graph to demonstrate differences in disease progression with time. (Courtesy of Manson Publishing. Schaer M. *Clinical Medicine of the Dog and Cat.* 2nd edn. fig. 1367, p. 684.)

- Treatment goals:
  - ○ alleviate discomfort.
  - ○ retard disease development (**1.29**).
  - ○ restore near-normal function.
  - ○ minimize joint instabilities.

While an extremely useful modality, the radiological examination has the following limitations:
- Bony lesions take time to develop.
- Permanent cartilage damage precedes radiographic changes.
- Changes with septic arthritis take 14–17 days.
- Nonerosive immune-mediated arthropathies may show no bony lesions.
- Osteoarthritic changes may obscure changes associated with neoplasia or infectious causes of joint disease.
- Severity of clinical signs cannot be predicted from radiographs.

Although the diagnosis of OA is not always obvious, especially in the early phases, the most consistent findings include altered activity, gait abnormalities, joint pain, joint effusion, and restricted joint ROM.

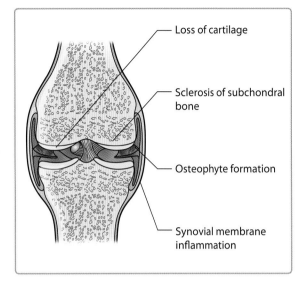

1.28 Location of degenerative joint disease characteristic changes.

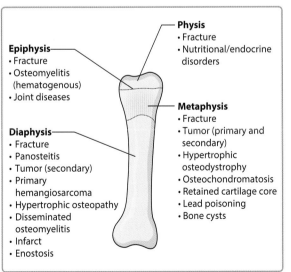

1.27 Diagram of bone disease location. (Courtesy of Manson Publishing. Schaer M. *Clinical Medicine of the Dog and Cat*. 2nd edn. fig. 1368, p. 685.)

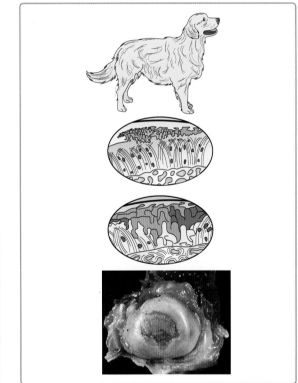

1.29 Degenerative joint disease progresses (top to bottom) from fibrillation of the hyaline cartilage, to deep crevassing, to loss of hyaline cartilage and replacement with inferior (structure and function) fibrocartilage, or loss of fibrocartilage and eburnation of subchondral bone.

Table 1.4 Diagnosis of OA

Method	Features		
History Distant observation	Assess body conformation Note decrease in weight bearing or altered limb motion Observe for trembling while standing Note asymmetric joint or soft tissue swelling Discern muscle atrophy Notice digit and joint alignment (dogs with tarsocrural OCD tend to be straight legged)		
Gait assessment	Chronic lameness often 'disappears' in the exam room Gait is observed at a walk and trot, with the dog moving towards and away from the observer, as well as from the side Observe ambulation on various surfaces, as well as on inclines and stairs 'Covert lameness' may become apparent with tight circles or stair climbing Gait abnormalities may include:	Shortened stride Toe-in/toe-out Stumbling Audible click Leg criss-crossing Dragging toenails Limb circumduction Ataxia Head bob Asymmetric pelvic motion Weakness Hypermetria Vocalization	
Standing palpation	Examine the contralateral limb simultaneously, looking for asymmetry from:	Trauma Degenerative changes Inflammation Congenital defects Neoplasia	
	Palpate for:	Swelling Heat Malalignment Crepitus Muscle atrophy	
Recumbent examination Diagnostic aids	Arthroscopy Diagnostic imaging		Radiography Fluoroscopy Ultrasonography Nuclear medicine Computed tomography Magnetic resonance imaging
	Routine laboratory evaluation		Hematology Biochemical profile Urinalysis Arthrocentesis Microbiologic examination Serology

REFERENCES

1 Hadler N. Why does the patient with osteoarthritis hurt? In: Brandt KD, Doherty M, Lohmander LS (eds). *Osteoarthritis*. Oxford University Press, New York, 1998, pp. 255–61.

2 Kellgren JH, Samuel EP. The sensitivity and innervation of the articular capsule. *J Bone Joint Surg* 1950;**4**:193–205.

3 Reimann I, Christensen SB. A histological demonstration of nerves in subchondral bone. *Acta Orthop Scand* 1977;**48**:345–52.

4 Arnoldi CC, Djurhuus JC, Heerfordt J, *et al.* Intraosseous phlebography, intraosseus pressure measurements, and 99mTc polyphosphate scintigraphy in patients with painful conditions in the hip and knee. *Acta Orthop Scand* 1980;**51**:19–28.

5 Suter PF. Normal radiographic anatomy and radiographic examination. In: Suter PF. *Thoracic Radiography: Thoracic Disease of the Dog and Cat*. Wettswil, Switzerland, 1984, p. 2.

6 Moskowitz R. Bone remodeling in osteoarthritis: subchondral and osteophytic responses. *Osteoarthr Cartilage* 1999;**7**:323–4.

7 Cicuttini FM, Baker J, Hart DJ, *et al.* Association of pain with radiological changes in different compartments and views of the knee joint. *Osteoarthr Cartilage* 1996;**4**:143–7.

8 Leach RE, Gregg T, Siber FJ. Weight-bearing radiograpy in osteoarthritis of the knee. *Radiology* 1970;**97**:265–8.

9 Brandt KD, Fife RS, Braunstein EM, *et al.* Radiographic grading of the severity of knee osteoarthritis: relation of the Killgren and Lawrence grade to a grade based on joint space narrowing, and correlation with arthroscopic evidence of articular cartilage degeneration. *Arthritis Rheumatol* 1991;**34**:1381–6.

10 Morgan JP. Radiological pathology and diagnosis of degenerative joint disease in the stifle joint of the dog. *J Small Anim Pract* 1969;**10**:541–4.

11 Lozier SM, Menard M. Arthrocentesis and synovial fluid analysis. In: Bojrab MJ (ed). *Current Techniques in Small Animal Surgery*, edn 4. Williams & Wilkins, Baltimore, 1998, p. 1057.

Chapter 2

Osteoarthritis: the Disease

DEFINITION

Osteoarthritis (OA) can be defined as a disorder of articular joints characterized by deterioration of articular cartilage; osteophyte formation and bone remodeling; pathology of periarticular tissues including synovium, subchondral bone, muscle, tendon, and ligament; and a low-grade, nonpurulent inflammation of variable degree. OA is differentiated from rheumatoid arthritis (RA), which is the classic example of a primary immune-mediated systemic condition characterized by bone destruction and articular cartilage erosion. RA is a more destructive, progressive, and debilitating condition than OA. Other forms of arthritis should be similarly differentiated from OA.

OA is not a single disease, and is often misperceived as a disease of only cartilage. It is a disease condition of the entire diarthrodial joint, including the articular (hyaline) cartilage, synovial membrane, synovial fluid, subchondral bone, and surrounding supporting structures (muscles and ligaments). The joint can be considered as an 'organ' where all components of the joint are affected by the disease process.

OA and degenerative joint disease (DJD) are synonyms; these two terms, and arthritis, arthrosis, rheumatism, and others, are often used interchangeably and incorrectly. Historically recognized as 'noninflammatory', OA is now realized to be an inflammatory condition, but the inflammation is not classically mediated by increased white blood cells in the synovial fluid as in other types of arthritis[1]. OA is associated with destruction and loss of cartilage, remodeling of bone, and intermittent inflammation. Changes in subchondral bone, synovium, and ligaments are detectable at an early stage, and initially an increase in cartilage matrix synthesis occurs concurrently with increased degradation. Synovial and cartilage-derived proteases are major players in cartilage matrix degradation, with matrix metalloproteinases (MMPs) and aggrecanases seemingly key catabolic agents. The vicious catabolic/anabolic cycle of OA is certainly not yet comprehensively understood. Although cartilage assuredly has the potential for endogenous repair, damage may become irreversible when compensation is exhausted or the imbalance between anabolic and catabolic processes is too great.

The pathologic changes that occur in the arthritic joint result in disability and clinical signs of pain. It is a complex condition involving multiple biochemical and biomechanical interactions (**2.1**). Often termed DJD, OA can be classified by the joint involved and whether it is primary or secondary. It appears to be mechanically driven but chemically mediated, with endogenous attempts at aberrant repair.

Prevalence in dogs

Osteoarthritis affects more than 80% of Americans over age 55 years[2] and approximately 1 in 5 adult dogs in the USA[3]. It is the number one cause of chronic pain in dogs, and approximately 10–12 million dogs in the USA show signs of OA. The 'average' veterinary practice sees approximately 45 arthritic dogs per month, 21% of which are considered 'severe', 38% are considered 'moderate', and 41% are considered 'mild' as assessed by their clinical presentation[4]. The demographics of dogs with OA are broad-reaching. Although the condition tends to be over-represented in older, heavy dogs, it can be a clinical problem in any dog. The 'poster child' for OA in dogs is the middle-aged to older (>4 years), large breed (>50 lb [>22.5 kg]) dog that is overweight to obese. OA is often secondary to either abnormal forces on normal joints (e.g. trauma, instability) or normal forces on abnormal joints (e.g. dysplasias, developmental disorders). In the case of obesity, which is often seen in older dogs, abnormal stress on the joints is accentuated.

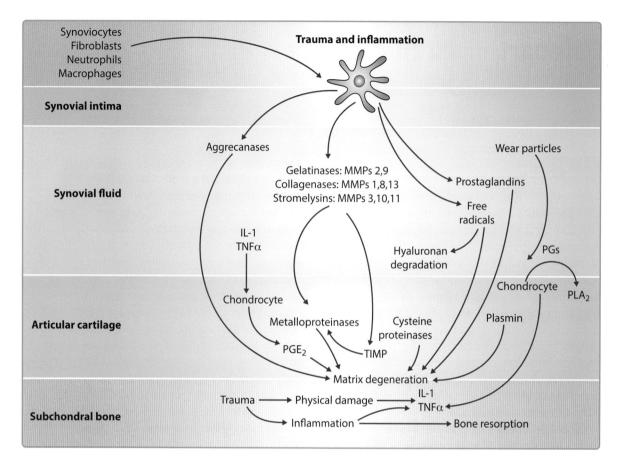

2.1 Osteoarthritis is a disease of the total joint ('organ') involving multiple biochemical and biomechanical interactions. IL: interleukin; MMP: matrix metalloproteinase; PLA: phospholipase A; PG: prostaglandin; TIMP: tissue inhibiting metalloproteinase.

Prevalence in cats

Almost 40% of American families own companion animals, comprising an estimated 72 million dogs and 82 million cats[5]. Cats, being light and agile, can compensate for fairly severe orthopedic disease, including musculoskeletal conditions such as OA. They are noted for hiding signs of lameness in the veterinarian's office, and observing the gait of cats is challenging, hindering the evaluation of lameness. Clinical signs of chronic pain at home, as reported by owners, include change of attitude (e.g. grumpy, slowing down) and disability (decreased grooming, missing the litter box on occasion, and inability to jump onto counters or furniture), rather than overt signs of lameness. Prevalence of radiographic signs of feline DJD ranges from 22% to 90% of investigated

populations[6–8]. Freire et al. have reported that 74% of 100 cats selected randomly from a database of 1640 cats in a single practice had DJD somewhere in the skeleton[9]. Freire et al. have also reported that radiographic appearance does not accurately predict whether or not feline joints show lesions associated with DJD[10]. In the latter report, 31 of 64 joints (elbow, hip, stifle, and hock) assessed from eight postmortem, euthanized animal shelter cats had radiographic signs of DJD. The absence of osteophytes did not predict normal-appearing cartilage, with 35 joints showing no radiographic osteophytes, but showing macroscopic cartilage lesions. There was no agreement between cartilage damage and the presence of sclerosis in the radiographs. In stifle, hock, and hip joints, no sclerosis was identified, even in those joints with moderate and severe cartilage damage. The best correlations and agreements between radiographic osteophyte score and macroscopic osteophyte score were in the elbow and hip. In the elbow, moderate cartilage damage was present before sclerosis was identified in the radiographs, and only mild sclerosis was identified in joints with severe cartilage damage.

These data, together with other published observations[6–8] suggest the prevalence of musculoskeletal disease (OA) in cats is much higher than most clinicians would predict. In turn, this might suggest that empirical treatment of a clinic's feline patient population (especially 'senior' cats) may yield improved quality of life (QOL) in as high as 90% of the patients. A caveat to this premise is conviction that a feline patient actually has a compromised QOL, and how that might be validated.

JOINT STRUCTURES

Proteoglycans comprise most of the extracellular matrix that is not collagen and make up 22–38% of the dry weight of adult articular cartilage[11]. The common glycosaminoglycans of articular cartilage are chondroitin sulfate, keratan sulfate, and dermatan sulfate. They are chains of variable length made up of repeating disaccharide subunits covalently attached to a protein core (**2.2**).

Subchondral bone is a thin layer of bone that joins hyaline cartilage with cancellous bone supporting the bony plate. The undulating nature of the osteochondral junction allows shear stresses to be converted into potentially less damaging compressive forces on the subchondral bone. The subchondral/cancellous region has been found to be approximately 10 times more deformable than cortical bone, and plays a major role in the distribution of forces across a joint[12]. Compliance of subchondral bone to applied joint forces allows congruity of joint surfaces for increasing the contact area of load distribution, thereby reducing peak loading and potential damage to cartilage[13]. Cartilage itself makes a poor shock absorber; however, subchondral bone well serves such a role.

Synovial fluid is frequently referred to as a dialysate of plasma, in that it contains electrolytes and small molecules in proportions similar to plasma. The release of inflammatory mediators results in increased permeability of synovial vasculature[14]. This results in increased synovial fluid protein content, with disturbance of the normal oncotic balance and increased synovial fluid volume.

The joint capsule can be divided into three strata, given various nomenclature, but the most commonly accepted refer to the synovium as the synovial lining (intima) and subsynovial layers, with the term joint capsule referring to the fibrous

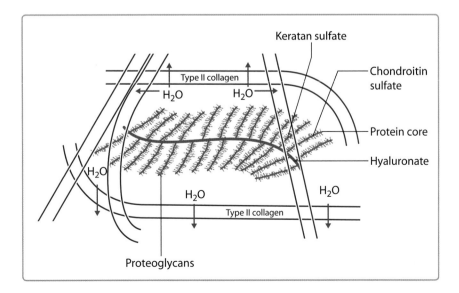

2.2 Cartilage integrity is maintained by the proteoglycan–hyaluronate aggregates. The collagen network retains its stiffness due to the outward pressure of water molecules held in the cartilage by the osmotic attraction of these aggregates.

tissue surrounding the joint. Within the synovial intima (usually only one to two cell layers thick) reside type A synoviocytes (macrophage-like in function) and type B synoviocytes (producing hyaluronan; also capable of producing degradative enzymes). The subsynovial layer is vascular, neural, and allows independent movement of the synovial membrane from the fibrous joint capsule. The tough fibrous layer contributes to physical stability of the joint. The fibrocartilaginous menisci are considered extensions of the joint capsule, although they are not covered by the synovial lining layer. Menisci function to enhance bone-to-bone conformation and grant the joint stability. They do not serve as 'shock absorbers', that is the role of subchondral bone.

The joint capsule plays a major role in OA, as changes in the synovium precede changes in the articular cartilage[15]. Articular cartilage receives its nutrients and clears its waste products by movement of fluid under the influence of weight bearing. This is analogous to the movement of water in and out of a sponge being squeezed while immersed within a bucket of water. Synovial lining macrophages phagocytize proteoglycans and collagen fragments released from diseased cartilage into the synovial fluid. This stimulates the synoviocytes to produce cytokines and MMPs, which, under the influence of weight bearing, are forced back into the cartilage matrix to further perpetuate the process of degradation[16]. Under the influence of prostaglandin E_2 (PGE_2) and other proinflammatory mediators, the villous synovium hypertrophies to a most vivid arthroscopically observed synovitis. Fibrosis and thickening of the more peripheral joint capsule result in a decreased range of motion and pain, clinically seen as patient stiffness.

INFLAMMATION IN OA

Inflammation in joints causes peripheral sensitization, with an upregulation of primary afferent neuron sensitivity, and also central sensitization, with hyperexcitability of nociceptive neurons in the central nervous system[17]. Inflammatory mediators (**2.3**) play a role either by directly activating high-threshold receptors or, more commonly, by sensitizing nociceptive neurons to subsequent daily stimuli. Damaged joints and sensory nervous system interactions may not only produce pain, but may actually influence the course of the disease (**2.4**).

Noteworthy to general small animal practice today is early (<6 months of age) neutering. The impetus for this widespread practice in the USA is presumably pet population control and the impression that mammary and prostate cancers are prevented and aggressive male behaviour is suppressed compared to those neutered later. Impact of this practice was revealed by Hart *et al.* in observing the long-term effects of neutering Labrador retrievers and golden retrievers[18]. In golden retrievers, neutering at <6 months of age increased the incidence of joint disorders (hip dysplasia and cruciate disease) to 4–5 times that of intact dogs. In Labrador retrievers (where about 5% of gonadally intact males and females had one or more joint disorders), neutering at <6 months doubled the incidence of one or more joint disorders in both sexes. Many European countries avoid neutering altogether. These observations illustrate the impact of sex hormones on OA and suggest an obligation clinicians have is to inform clients of the consequences associated with neutering.

Osteoarthritis overlays a more specific focus when considering DJD associated with the cranial

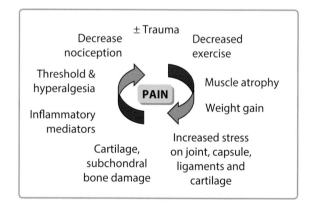

2.3 Osteoarthritis (OA) appears to be mechanically driven, but chemically mediated, with endogenous attempts at aberrant repair. Although clinically apparent, the vicious catabolic/anabolic cycle of OA is not yet comprehensively understood; however, recent evidence suggests inflammation may be at the genesis of this degradative process.

2.4 Degradation and synthesis of cartilage matrix components are related to the release of mediators by chondrocytes, ligamentocytes (fibroblasts), and synoviocytes; including the cytokines interleukin (IL)-1β and tumor necrosis factor (TNF), nitric oxide, prostaglandins (PG) and growth factors. A minor injury could start the disease process in a less resistant environment, whereas in other individuals, the joint may be able to compensate for a greater insult. Damage may become irreversible when compensation fails. MMP: matrix metalloproteinase; NSAID: nonsteroidal anti-inflammatory drug; COX: cyclo-oxygenase; iNOS: inducible nitric oxide synthase; PSGAG: polysulfated glycosaminoglycan; HA: hyaluronic acid.

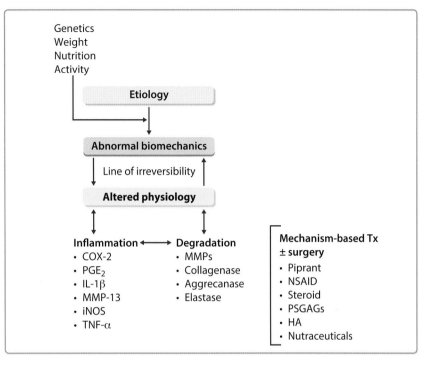

cruciate ligament (CCL). Although acute CCL rupture can occur with trauma, the majority of ruptures result from chronic degenerative changes within the ligament[19,20]. Recent work clearly shows that stifle arthritis precedes the development of CCL rupture and associated stifle instability in the majority of affected dogs (**2.5**).

A central hypothesis regarding the initial mechanism that leads to CCL disease is activation of synovial immune responses and development of a chronic synovitis that promotes CCL degeneration – as ligament nutrition and metabolism are related to synovial fluid physiology[24]. Studies support the proposal that persistent synovitis and development of an inflammatory arthritis are likely significant factors promoting degenerative rupture of the CCL[25]. Pro-inflammatory cytokines, synthesized in both cartilage and the synovium (**2.6, 2.7**), potentiate the cascade of biologically active substances that contribute to the degradation of the joint[26].

Nitric oxide (NO) is an important mediator in both physiologic and pathophysiologic pathways. It is believed to be mainly catabolic in joint physiology.

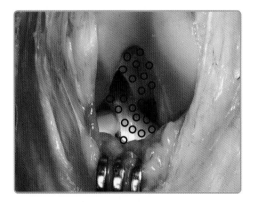

2.5 The cruciate ligaments are covered by a fold of synovial membrane and although they have an intra-articular position, they are extrasynovial[21]. Scanning microscopy reveals the presence of many small holes in the enveloping membrane (exaggerated here), allowing infiltration of the cruciate ligaments by synovial fluid and its contents[22]. These 'pores' allow the movement of macromolecules, including immune complexes. Cruciate ligament metabolism is, therefore, closely related to changes in synovial fluid[23].

NO is generated through the activation of inducible nitric oxide synthase (iNOS), which is calcium-independent, and thereby long-lasting, which generates large amounts of NO over an extended period of time[29]. NO inhibits the synthesis of proteoglycans and collagen in cartilage culture and up-regulates the synthesis of MMPs that are typically kept in check by tissue-inhibiting metalloproteinases (TIMPs). NO is also known to mediate apoptosis in joint tissues, as well as mediate the expression of proinflammatory cytokines such as interleukin (IL)-18 and IL-1 converting enzyme[30, 31].

Matrix metalloproteinases are a group of endopeptidases ubiquitous to almost every inflammatory disease state. A homeostatic balance between MMPs and TIMPs controls tissue remodeling and synthesis[32]. Within the joint, MMPs are produced by synovial cells, cartilage, ligamentocytes

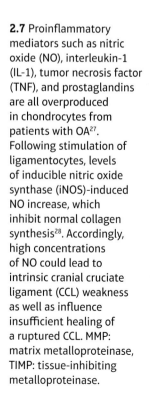

2.6 As the joint is loaded and unloaded by weight bearing, inflammatory mediators and degradative agents from both the synovial intima lining and cartilage are inter-mingled: analogous to a sponge being squeezed and released. This activity enhances the distribution of catabolic mediators.

2.7 Proinflammatory mediators such as nitric oxide (NO), interleukin-1 (IL-1), tumor necrosis factor (TNF), and prostaglandins are all overproduced in chondrocytes from patients with OA[27]. Following stimulation of ligamentocytes, levels of inducible nitric oxide synthase (iNOS)-induced NO increase, which inhibit normal collagen synthesis[28]. Accordingly, high concentrations of NO could lead to intrinsic cranial cruciate ligament (CCL) weakness as well as influence insufficient healing of a ruptured CCL. MMP: matrix metalloproteinase, TIMP: tissue-inhibiting metalloproteinase.

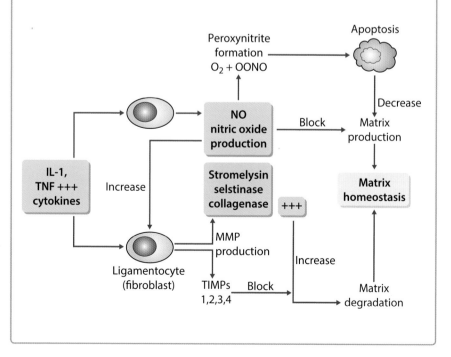

(fibroblasts), and leukocytes. Based mainly on their substrate they can be characterized as collagenases, gelatinases, stromelysins, and membrane-type.

A listing of destructive and pathologic factors in OA is extensive; however, major players include: cyclo-oxygenase-2 (COX-2), PGE_2, IL-1β, MMP-13, iNOS, tumor necrosis factor (TNF)-α, and nuclear factor kappa B (NF-κB) (*Table 2.1*, **2.8**). COX-2 is an isozyme of the arachidonic acid (AA) pathway which gives rise to several eicosanoids associated with pain and inflammation–pathologic manifestations of the AA pathway. PGE_2 is an end-product of COX-2 metabolism, most frequently recognized for its clinical result in pain and inflammation. Interleukin-1β and TNF-α are the primary cytokines mediating the pathogenesis of OA. Studies have shown that abnormally high levels of IL-1β and TNF-α are present in the synovial fluid, synovium, and cartilage tissue of OA patients[33,34]. *In vitro* studies have shown that both IL-1β and TNF-α stimulate secretion of prostaglandins and increase the activity of matrix-degrading proteinases such

COX-2
PGE_2
IL-1β
MMP-13
iNOS
TNF-α

2.8 There are a number of inflammatory mediators associated with OA and which may contribute to cranial cruciate ligament (CCL) failure as well as pain. Some of the more influential are: cyclo-oxygenase-2, prostaglandin E_2, interleukin-1 (IL-1), matrix metalloproteinase (MMP-13), nitric oxide (from inducible nitric oxide synthase), tumor necrosing factor-α (TNF-α) and NF-κB (nuclear factor kappa-light-chain-enhancer of activated B cells). MMP: matrix metalloproteinase; COX-2: cyclo-oxygenase 2; iNOS: inducible nitric oxide synthase.

Table 2.1 Major inflammatory mediators of osteoarthritis

Inflammatory mediator	Degradative activity
COX-2	Cyclo-oxygenase-2 gives rise to destructive and inflammatory eicosanoids
PGE_2	Prostaglandin E_2 is a major enzyme in the arachidonic acid pathway leading to the pathologic features of pain and inflammation
IL-1β	Interleukin-1β induces COX-2 with resultant central nervous system hypersensitivity. Both IL-1α and IL-1β possess strong proinflammatory effects
MMP-13	Matrix metalloproteinase-13 (collagenase 3) cleaves type II collagen
iNOS	Inducible nitric oxide (NO) synthase leads to increased synthesis of NO, associated with cartilage degradation, inhibition of matrix synthesis, and chondrocyte apoptosis
TNF-α	Tumor necrosis factor-α stimulates prostaglandin secretion and increases activity of matrix-degrading proteinases as well as regulating immune cells
NF-kB	Nuclear factor kappa B controls transcription of DNA and can be responsible for cytokine production and cell survival

as collagenase, gelatinase, proteoglycanase, stromelysin, and plasminogen activator[35,36]. Although IL-1β is physiologically more potent than TNF-α, animal studies suggest the two cytokines act synergistically to stimulate cartilage degradation–exceeding the damage observed with either cytokine alone[37]. IL-1β and TNF-α also induce the synthesis of the COX-2 and iNOS enzymes. This leads to elevated levels of PGE$_2$ and NO: up-regulating cartilage degradation, inhibition of matrix synthesis, and chondrocyte apoptosis[38,39,40,41]. Interleukins (IL-1) also stimulate fibroblasts to produce collagen types I and III. This may contribute to fibrosis of the joint capsule in OA patients[42].

MMP-13 (collagenase 3) is secreted as an inactive protein, which is activated when cleaved by extracellular proteinases. MMP-13 plays a key role in degradation and remodeling of host extracellular matrix proteins, including degradation of type II collagen. By cleaving the triple helix of type II collagen and core protein of the aggrecan, it induces major irreversible damage to the cartilage matrix structure. In doing so, the biophysical properties of cartilage are modified, reducing its resilience to the abnormal biomechanical forces present in OA. MMP-13 has been shown to be preferentially increased in the deep zone of cartilage (perpendicular zone), and is considered a major catabolic factor in that zone as well as in OA lesional areas[43–45].

Under the influence of iNOS stimulation by various cytokines, OA cartilage produces an excessive amount of NO. It is proposed that NO contributes to the development of arthritic lesions by inhibiting the synthesis of cartilage matrix macromolecules and by inducing chondrocyte death, which could further contribute to the reduction of extracellular matrix in OA[46,47,48,49,50,51]. NO is also known to reduce the synthesis of the IL-1 receptor antagonist in chondrocytes, a process possibly responsible for the enhanced IL-1β effect on these cells. Finally, diffusion of NO from the superficial layer of cartilage (tangential zone) to the deeper zone may also contribute to increasing the level of MMP-13 synthesis at the deeper level[52,53]. Overproduction of cytokines, such as TNF-α, stimulates cartilage matrix degradation by inhibiting the production of proteoglycans and type II collagen while up-regulating the production of matrix-degrading enzymes such as MMPs[54]. Such cytokines also upregulate the expression of COX-2 and iNOS: leading to increased synthesis of PGE$_2$ and NO[55,56].

NF-κB (nuclear factor kappa-light-chain-enhancer of activated B cells), found in almost all animal cell types, is a protein complex that controls transcription of DNA. NF-κB plays a key role in regulating the immune response to infection. Incorrect regulation of NF-κB has been linked to cancer, inflammatory, and autoimmune diseases, septic shock, viral infection, and improper immune development. In brief, NF-κB can be understood to be a protein responsible for cytokine production and cell survival.

In unstimulated cells, the NF-κB dimers are sequestered in the cytoplasm by a family of inhibitors, called IκBs (inhibitor of κB). The IκB proteins mask nuclear localization signals of NF-κB proteins and keep them sequestered in an inactive state in the cytoplasm. Activation of the NF-κB is initiated by a signal-induced degradation of IκB proteins. This occurs primarily via activation of a kinase called the IκB kinase. With the degradation of IκB, the NF-κB complex is then freed to enter the nucleus where it can 'turn on' the expression of specific genes that have DNA-binding sites for NF-κB nearby. The activation of these genes by NF-κB leads to the given physiological response, e.g. an inflammatory or immune response. Due to its orchestrating role in inflammation, NF-κB is often referred to as the 'switch' that turns on the inflammatory pathway. Many natural products (including anti-oxidants) that have been promoted to have anti-cancer and anti-inflammatory activity have been shown to inhibit NF-κB, and extracts from a number of herbs and dietary plants have been shown to be efficient inhibitors of NF-κB activation *in vitro*.

Recognizing influential inflammatory mediators as major players in the pathogenesis of OA (with resultant influence on CCL disease) has made them targets for disease prophylaxis and treatment[57].

The inflammatory component of OA is more prevalent at different phases of the disease. The synovial fluid of most OA patients shows mildly increased numbers of mononuclear cells and increased levels of immunoglobulins and complement. The synovial membrane shows signs of chronic inflammation including hyperplasia of the lining with infiltration of inflammatory cells. Inflammation likely plays an important role in the painful symptoms of OA[58].

OA frequently results in osteophyte formation. Osteophytes are a central core of bone that blend in with the subchondral bone (**2.9**). They are covered by hyaline and fibrocartilage and are formed by a process similar to enchondral ossification[59]. Although they may occur centrally in the joint, they are most frequently found at the junction of the synovium, perichondrium, and periosteum[60]. Chondrophyte and osteophyte growth results in elevation and stretching of richly innervated periosteum which is also a common origin of expansile bone tumor pain.

The term enthesiophytes refers to bony proliferations found at the insertion of ligaments, tendons, and capsule to bone. Ligaments and muscles surrounding the OA joint contribute to the pain of OA. Although ligamentous neuroreceptors serve mainly to determine spatial orientation of the joint, or joint position awareness, tissue stretch also incites pain. Muscle weakness accompanying OA is also associated with pain and disability. Stimulation of neuroreceptors within the damaged OA joint can stimulate a reflex arc resulting in constant stimulation of muscle tissue. Muscle spasm and muscle fatigue may greatly contribute to the pain of OA. Mild muscle trauma likely results in the release of inflammatory mediators, sensitizing muscle nociceptors to further mechanical stimulation. Local tenderness often results from the release of inflammatory mediators such as bradykinin and PGE_2. Nociceptors are found in muscle, fascia, and tendons, and since afferent nerve fibers from muscle distribute over a relatively large region of the dorsal spinal horn, poor localization of muscle pain is common.

Pain from meniscal tearing and disruption comes from stimulation of joint capsule pain receptors and perhaps from stimulation of C fibers in the outer one-third of the meniscus[61].

THE 'PAIN PATHWAY'

There is no pain pathway! Pain is the result of a complex signaling network. The cognition of pain, like cognition in general, requires sophisticated neurologic hardware. The physiologic component of pain is termed nociception, which consists of the processes of transduction, transmission, and modulation of neural signals generated in response to a noxious stimulus. When carried to completion in the conscious animal, nociception results in pain. Simplistically, the pain track can be understood as a three-neuron chain, with the first-order neuron originating in the periphery and projecting to the spinal cord, the second-order neuron ascending the spinal cord, and the third-order neuron projecting to the cerebral cortex. In actuality, the track involves a network of branches and communications with other sensory neurons and descending inhibitory neurons from the midbrain that modulate afferent transmission of noxious stimuli.

The process begins with the conversion by nociceptors of mechanical, chemical, or thermal energy into electrical impulses. These nociceptors exist as free nerve endings of primary afferent neurons, and have considerably higher stimulus thresholds for activation than thermoreceptors or low-threshold mechanoreceptors active under ambient conditions. Within the dorsal horn, the communication of afferent nociceptive information between various neurons occurs via chemical signaling, mediated by excitatory and inhibitory amino acids and neuropeptides that are produced, stored, and released in the terminals of afferent nerve fibers and dorsal horn neurons. It is here in the dorsal horn that the afferent nociceptive impulse lives or dies, and is modulated by various integrative influences.

The descending modulatory system can be described as having four tiers: 1) the cortical and thalamic structures; 2) the periaqueductal gray matter of the midbrain; 3) the rostral medulla and pons of the brainstem; and 4) the medullary and spinal cord dorsal horn. Again, the spinal cord is the site of most active modulation. Dense concentrations of γ-aminobutyric acid, glycine, serotonin,

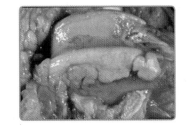

2.9 Osteophytes are characteristic of degenerative joint disease and are formed by a process similar to endochondral ossification.

norepinephrine, and the endogenous opioid pep-tides (enkephalins, endorphins, and dynorphins) have been identified in dorsal horn neurons, and all produce inhibitory effects on nociceptive transmission. It is now apparent that a single neuron may be influenced by many neurotransmitters, that each neurotransmitter may have numerous actions in a given region, and that multiple neurotransmitters may exist within a single neuron. Details of the processing of nociception to pain are beyond the scope of this work, but may be sourced elsewhere[62].

It is important to note that the pain response is not confined to the nervous system. Pain induces both segmental and suprasegmental reflex responses which result in: increased sympathetic tone; vasoconstriction; increased system vascular resistance; increased cardiac output through increases in both stroke volume and heart rate; increased myocardial work through increases in metabolic rate and oxygen consumption, decreased gastrointestinal and urinary tone; and increased skeletal muscle tone. Endocrine responses include increased secretion of adrenocorticotrophic hormone, cortisol, antidiuretic hormone, growth hormone, cyclic adenosine monophosphate, catecholamines, renin, angiotensin II, aldosterone, glucagons, and IL-1, with concomitant decreases in insulin and testosterone secretion, i.e. the classic stress response.

Identifying and scoring pain in the arthritic animal

As a rule-of-thumb, any change in behavior can signal pain. However, the most reliable indicator of pain is response to an analgesic. Physiologic parameters, including heart rate, respiratory rate, blood pressure, and temperature, are not consistent or reliable indicators of pain. Various acute pain assessment measures have been used by researchers to quantify pain. These include verbal rating scales (VRS), simple descriptive scales (SDS), numeric rating scales (NRS), and visual analog scales (VAS), all of which have their limitations. Historical limitations of scales used to assess pain have included assessment of pain on intensity alone. Such limitations have led to development of multidimensional scales, taking into account the sensory and affective qualities of pain in addition to its intensity. The Glasgow Pain Scale[63] is such a multidimensional scheme, and

although it is detailed, its on-going refinement may result in greater utilization. Currently, there are no validated 'scales' to assess chronic pain. Several investigators have suggested exploring this area of interest through the creation of novel questionnaires as an instrument for measuring chronic pain in dogs through its impact on health-related quality of life (HRQL)[64–66].

Expanding on the value of owner assessment, a client-specific outcome measures scheme has been developed for pets based on the Cincinnati Orthopedic Disability Index (CODI) for people[67]. In this scheme, five very specific problems related to OA are identified; these are recorded, and the intensity of the problem is monitored as treatment progresses. Because the questions are very specific to the individual animal in its environment, this measurement system appears to be very sensitive.

An example of a very specific questionnaire used at North Carolina State University Comparative Pain Research Laboratory to assess pain associated with clinical OA in cats is seen in **2.10**. Activity or behavior that is suspected to be altered as a result of the pain, specific to the animal and its home environment, is defined. Activities are graded before the start of treatment and after analgesic treatment is started. A left shift corresponds to pain relief.

MORPHOLOGICAL CHANGES WITH OA

The tangentially oriented collagen fibrils of the superficial cartilage zone, along with relatively low proteoglycan content, have the greatest ability to withstand high tensile stresses, thereby resisting deformation and distributing shearing load more evenly over the joint surface (**2.11**). Loss of this superficial layer, as occurs in the early stages of cartilage fibrillation of OA, alters the biomechanical properties of the articular cartilage. One of the first changes of OA, recognized microscopically, is fibrillation of the superficial cartilage layer[68]. Fibrillation occurs as a flaking of the superficial cartilage layers, following the course of collagen fibrils that run parallel to the joint surface. Once the integrity of this outer layer of cartilage is lost by the progression of fibrillation, abnormal stresses give rise to fissures into the deeper layers. These fissures develop in a vertical plane, again following the orientation of

Problems in mobility related to osteoarthritis in your cat	No problem	A little problematic	Quite problematic	Severely problematic	Impossible
1 Jumping onto sofa		▽	✓		
2 Jumping onto kitchen counter			▽		✓
3 Walking up steps on back deck	▽		✓		
4 Jumping on bed	▽				✓
5 Using litter tray	▽	✓			

✓ Start of treatment   ▽ After treatment

2.10 Client-specific outcome measure questionnaire on activity.

2.11 Hyaline cartilage comprises three different zones, based on chondrocyte organization, collagen fiber orientation, and proteoglycan distribution. The tangentially oriented collagen fibrils of the superficial zone have the greatest ability to withstand high tensile stresses, thereby resisting deformation and distributing load more evenly over the joint surface.

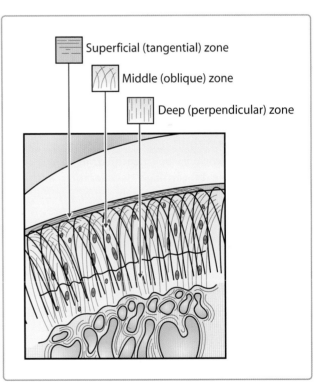

Superficial (tangential) zone

Middle (oblique) zone

Deep (perpendicular) zone

midzone collagen fibrils. Such fissures can extend to the subchondral bone. Concurrently, chondrocytes become larger and begin to cluster. The release of free cartilage fragments initiates a synovitis as they are phagocytized by type A synoviocytes[69].

Synovitis

It is proposed that the chondrocyte is the most active source of degradative protease production; however, this is stimulated primarily by cytokines and leukotrienes produced by the synovium[70]. Yet it appears that synovitis alone is insufficient as the sole etiology of OA, and that physical trauma is also necessary[71]. Models that reduce joint inflammation slow the degeneration of articular cartilage. For example, strict hemostasis results in decreased development of degenerative articular change in a cruciate deficient model (i.e. producing less inflammatory stimulus), illustrating the importance of the synovium in the development of OA changes[72]. It is therefore logical to assume that intervention in the inflammatory process of OA may slow the disease process (**2.12**).

Joint capsule dynamics

Progressive alterations of the synovium include thickening of the synovial intima from one to two cell layers thick to three to four cell layers thick, development of synovial villi, and increased vascularity and infiltration of the subsynovial stroma by lymphocytes[73]. Apparently, changes in the synovium precede changes in the articular cartilage.

OA and joint instability

OA can, simplistically, be identified as consequential sequelae to cartilage degeneration and the persistent trigger from instability of a joint.

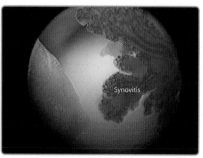

2.12 Arthroscopic view of synovitis, characterized by infiltration of the synovial membrane with inflammatory cells resulting in vascularization and hyperplasia of the synovium. Synovitis is believed to contribute to the development of pain, joint inflammation, and progression of osteoarthritis.

Surgically induced instability models of OA have been described in various animal species. Humans with a traumatic injury generally decrease use of the affected limb until restabilization has occurred. In animals, where restabilization has not occurred, the disease progression is usually much more rapid, making it much less amenable to therapeutic intervention[74,75]. Surgically induced models of OA, especially in rodents and rabbits, usually have rapid and severe cartilage degeneration after the instability is created and, generally, the greater the instability, the greater the lesion[76]. Surgical instability models of OA have been produced in rats, guinea pigs, rabbits, sheep, goats, and dogs[77-80].

The most frequently described canine model of OA-related joint degeneration is the cranial cruciate ligament transection (CCLT) model. Here, joint instability is the driving force in the development of degenerative features. Joint degeneration, as a result of acutely altered biomechanics, is perpetuated by inflammatory responses secondary to the inflammation from poor resistance to shear mechanical stress of hyaline cartilage and due to the ligament endings in the joint, triggering an inflammatory response[81-83]. In 53–74% of CCLT dogs, medial meniscal damage occurred[84], which, itself, is a driving force of joint degeneration[85]. Accordingly, the combination of CCLT and meniscal damage constitutes a robust destabilizing drive for the development of OA[86]. In the CCLT model, permanent instability in the knee joint is followed by degenerative changes in cartilage and changes in synovial tissue (representing secondary synovitis) that, over the course of several months, lead to canine OA[82]. Separating the two etiologies (instability and cartilage damage), the canine 'groove' model of OA has been proposed to exclude the influence of instability[87].

Though not objectively evaluated, it has long been assumed that capsular thickening in a CCL deficient canine knee functions to stabilize the joint over time[88-90]. The goal of reconstructive surgical methods should be not only to alleviate the existing instability of the unstable stifle joint, but also to mimic normal kinematics as closely as possible. Extracapsular suture techniques provide stifle joint stability through static neutralization of cranial drawer without alteration of stifle joint anatomy[91]. The tibial plateau leveling osteotomy has been used to provide dynamic stability to the stifle joint by alteration of the tibial plateau angle[92]. More recently, the tibial tuberosity advancement technique has been proposed to stabilize the stifle joint during weight bearing by neutralizing cranial tibial thrust[93,94].

Studies indicate that passive hip joint laxity is the primary risk factor for the development of DJD in dogs with hip dysplasia[95,96]. It is hypothesized that in some dogs, passive joint laxity is transformed into functional laxity during weight bearing, thereby exposing the cartilaginous surfaces of the joint to excessive stresses. Such stresses cause cartilage damage and microfracture, release of inflammatory mediators, and, ultimately, the changes associated with DJD. Functional laxity appears to be both necessary and sufficient for the development of DJD[97]. Surgical management of hip dysplasia may involve corrective osteotomies or arthroplasty techniques, all designed to improve joint congruency and stability. Total hip arthroplasty may be performed in adult dogs with chronically painful hips that cannot be treated satisfactorily by other methods.

As with the knee and hip, instability is considered a primary etiological factor in elbow dysplasia[98]. Elbow incongruity is the term used to describe poor alignment of the elbow joint surfaces. Two illustrative features are: 1) an abnormal shape of the ulnar trochlear notch; and 2) a step between the radius and ulna, caused by either a short radius or a short ulna. The suggestion is that both an elliptical notch and a step can cause increased local pressure within the joint, resulting in fragmentation at different locations, clinically recognized as ununited anconeal process (UAP), fragmented coronoid process (FCP), and osteochondritis dissecans (OCD) of the humeral condyle. Collectively, these lesions are referred to as 'elbow dysplasia'. Several surgical techniques have been proposed, and are currently under development, to restore joint congruity and improve function[99]. It has been proposed that incongruity worsens the prognosis after surgery to remove loose fragments[100], accounting for 30–40% of postoperative patients still showing lameness. Owing to the recognition that a 'satisfying' treatment for elbow dysplasia is still to be identified, homogenous tin-117m colloid (HTC) radiosynoviorthesis is being developed as a treatment option.

REFERENCES

1   Yuan GH, Masukp-Hongo K, Kato T, et al. Immunologic intervention in the pathogenesis of osteoarthritis. *Arthritis Rheumatol* 2003;**48**:602–11.

2   Kee CC. Osteoarthritis: manageable scourge of aging. *Nurs Clin North Am* 2000;**35**:199–208.

3   Pfizer Animal Health proprietary market research; survey of 200 veterinarians, 1996.

4   Rimadyl A&U Study, USA: 039 DRIM 197.

5   *US Pet Ownership and Demographics Sourcebook, AVMA*, 2007. (www.avma.org/ reference/ marketstats/ownership.asp).

6   Hardie EM, Roe SC, Martin FR. Radiographic evidence of degenerative joint disease in geriatric cats: 100 cases (1994–1997). *JAVMA* 2002;**220**:628–32.

7   Godfrey DR. Osteoarthritis in cats: a retrospective radiological study. *J Small Anim Pract* 2005;**46**:425–9.

8   Clarke SP, Mellor D, Clements DN, et al. Prevalence of radiographic signs of degenerative joint disease in a hospital population of cats. *Vet Record* 2005;**157**:793–9.

9   Freire M, Simpson W, Thomson A, et al. Cross-sectional study evaluating the radiographic prevalence of feline degenerative joint disease. 2008 ACVS Annual Meeting, San Diego, CA.

10 Freire M, Hash J, Lascelles BDX. Evaluation of postmortem radiological appearance versus macroscopic appearance of appendicular joints in cats. 2008 ACVS Annual Meeting, San Diego, CA.

11 Mankin HJ, Brandt KD. Pathogenesis of osteoarthritis. In: Kelly WN, Harris ED, Ruddy S, Sledge CB (eds). *Textbook of Rheumatology*, edn 5. WB Saunders, Philadelphia, 1997, p.1369.

12 Radin EL, Paul IL, Lowry M. A comparison of the dynamic force transmitting properties of subchondral bone and articular cartilage. *J Bone Joint Surg Am* 1970;**52**:444–56.

13 Radin EL, Paul IL. Does cartilage reduce skeletal impact loads? The relative force-attenuating properties of articular cartilage, synovial fluid, periarticular soft tissues, and bone. *Arthritis Rheumatol* 1970;**13**:139–44.

14 Simkin PA. Synovial physiology. In: Koopman

WJ (ed). *Arthritis and Allied Conditions*, edn 13. Williams & Wilkins, Baltimore, 1997, p. 193.

15 Lust G, Summers BA. Early, asymptomatic stage of degenerative joint disease in canine hip joints. *Am J Vet Res* 1981;**42**:1849–55.

16 Pelletier JP, Martel-Pelletier J, Ghandur-Mnaymneh L, *et al.* Role of synovial membrane inflammation in cartilage matrix breakdown in the Pond–Nuki dog model of osteoarthritis. *Arthritis Rheumatol* 1985;**28**:554–61.

17 Schaible HGT, Ebersberger A, Von Banchet GS. Mechanisms of pain in arthritis. *Ann NY Acad Sci* 2002;**966**:343–54.

18 Hart BL, Hart LA, Thigpen AP, *et al.* Long-term health effects of neutering dogs: comparison of Labrador Retrievers with Golden Retrievers. *Plos One*. July 2014, **9**,(7).

19 Vasseur PB, Pool RR, Arnoczky SP, *et al.* Correlative biomechanical and histologic study of the cranial cruciate ligament in dogs. *Am J Vet Res* 1985;**46**:1842–54.

20 Hayashi K, Frank JD, Dubinsky C, *et al.* Histologic changes in ruptured canine cranial cruciate ligament. *Vet Surg* 2003;**32**:269–77.

21 Arnoczky SP, Rubin RM, Marshall JL. Microvasculature of the cruciate ligaments and its response to injury. An experimental study in dogs. *J Bone Joint Surg Am* 1979;**61**:1221–9.

22 Kobayashi S, Baba H, Uchida K, *et al.* Microvascular system of anterior cruciate ligament in dogs. *J Orthop Res* 2006;**24**:1509–20.

23 Bari AS, Carter SD, Bell SC, *et al.* Anti-type II collagen antibody in naturally occurring canine joint diseases. *Br J Rheumatol* 1989;**28**:480–6.

24 Hayashi K, Muir P. Histology of cranial cruciate ligament rupture. In: Muir P (ed) *Advances in The Canine Cranial Cruciate Ligament*. Wiley-Blackwell, 2010, pp. 45–51.

25 Fujita Y, Hara Y, Ochi H, *et al.* Proinflammatory cytokine activities, matrix metalloproteinase-3 activity, and sulfated glycosaminoglycan content in synovial fluid of dogs with naturally acquired cranial cruciate ligament rupture. *Vet Surg* 2006;**35**:369–76.

26 Doom M, de Bruin T, de Rooster H, *et al.* Immunopathological mechanisms in dogs with rupture of the cranial cruciate ligament. *Vet Immunol Immunopathol* 2008;**125**:143–61.

27 Weinberg JB, Fermor B, Guilak F. Nitric oxide synthase and cyclooxygenase interactions in cartilage and meniscus: Relationships to joint physiology arthritis, and tissue repair. *Subcell Biochem* 2007;**42**:31–62.

28 Cao M, Stefanovic-RaciM, Georgescu HI, *et al.* Does nitric oxide help explain the differential healing capacity of the anterior cruciate, posterior cruciate, and medial collateral ligaments? *Am J Sports Med* 2000;**28**:176–82.

29 Weinberg JB, Fermor B, Guilak F. Nitric oxide synthase and cyclooxygenase interactions in cartilage and meniscus: Relationships to joint physiology arthritis, and tissue repair. *Subcell Biochem* 2007;**42**:31–62.

30 Gyger O, Botteron C, Doherr M, *et al.* Detection and distribution of apoptotic cell death in normal and diseased canine cranial cruciate ligaments. *Vet J* 2007;**174**:371–7.

31 Boileau C, Martel-Pelletier J, Moldovan F, *et al.* The in situ up-regulation of chondrocyte interleukin-1-converting enzyme and interleukin-18 levels in experimental osteoarthritis is mediated by nitric oxide. *Arthritis Rheum* 2002;**46**:2637–47.

32 Nagase H, Visse R, Murphy G. Structure and function of matrix metalloproteinases and TIMPs. *Cardiovasc Res* 2006;**69**:562–73.

33 Algner T, Kurz B, Fukui N, *et al.* Roles of chondrocytes in the pathogenesis of osteoarthritis. *Curr Opin Rheumatol* 2002;**14**:578–84.

34 Goldring SR, Goldring MB. The role of cytokines in cartilage matrix degeneration in osteoarthritis. *Clin Orthop* 2004;**427**(Suppl):S27–36.

35 Bunning RA, Russell RG. The effect of tumor necrosis factor alpha and gamma-interferon on the resorption of human articular cartilage and on the production of prostaglandin E and of caseinase activity by human articular chondrocytes. *Arthritis Rheum* 1989;**32**:780–4.

36 Campbell IK, Piccoli DS, Roberts MJ, *et al.* Effects of tumor necrosing factor alpha and beta on resorption of human articular cartilage and production of plasminogen activator by human articular chondrocytes. *Arthritis Rheum* 1990;**33**:542–52.

37 Henderson B, Pettipher ER. Arthritogenic actions of recombinant IL-1 and tumour necrosis factor

alpha in the rabbit: evidence for synergistic interactions between cytokines in vivo. *Clin Exp Immunol* 1989;**75**:306–10.

38 Goldring MB, Berenbaum F. Human chondrocyte culture models for studying cyclooxygenase expression and prostaglandin regulation of collagen gene expression. *Osteoarthr Cartilage* 1999;**7**(4):386–8.

39 Lotz M. The role of nitric oxide in articular cartilage damage. *Rheum Dis Clin North Am* 1999;**25**(2):269e82.

40 Notoya K, Jovanovic DV, Reboul P, *et al.* The induction of cell death in human osteoarthritis chondrocytes by nitric oxide is related to the production of prostaglandin E2 via the induction of cyclooxygenase-2. *J Immunol* 2000;**165**(6):3402–10.

41 Miwa M, Saura R, Hirata S, *et al.* Induction of apoptosis in bovine articular chondrocyte by prostaglandin E(2) through cAMP-dependent pathway. *Osteoarthr Cartilage* 2000;**8**(1):17–24.

42 Lotz M. Cytokines and their receptors. In: Koopman WJ (ed): *Arthritis and Allied Conditions*, edn 13. Williams & Wilkins, Baltimore, 1997, p. 2013.

43 Moldovan F, Pelletier JP, Hambor J, *et al.* Collagenase-3 (matrix metalloprotease 13) is preferentially localized in the deep layer of human arthritic cartilage in situ: in vitro mimicking effect by transforming growth factor beta. *Arthritis Rheum* 1997;**40**:1653–61.

44 Freemont AJ, Byers RJ, Taiwo YO, *et al.* In situ zymographic localisation of type II collagen degrading activity in osteoarthritic human articular cartilage. *Ann Rheum Dis* 1999;**58**:357–65.

45 Martel-Pelletier J, Welsch DJ, Pelletier JP. Metalloproteases and inhibitors in arthritic diseases. *Best Pract Res Clin Rheumatol* 2001;**15**(5):805–29.

46 Stefanovic-Racic M, Stadler J, Evans CH. Nitric oxide and arthritis. *Arthritis Rheum* 1993; **36**:1036–44.

47 Hickery MS, Palmer RM, Charles IG, *et al.* The role of nitric oxide in IL-1 and TNF alpha-induced inhibition of proteoglycan synthesis in human articular cartilage. *Trans Orthop Res Soc* 1994;**19**:77.

48 Taskiran D, Stefanovic-Racic M, Georgescu HI, *et al.* Nitric oxide mediates suppression of cartilage proteoglycan synthesis by interleukin-1. *Biochem Biophys Res Commun* 1994;**200**:142–8.

49 Järvinen TAH, Moilanen T, Järvinen TLN, *et al.* Nitric oxide mediates interleukin-1 induced inhibition of glycosaminoglycan synthesis in rat articular cartilage. *Mediators Inflamm* 1995;**4**:107–11.

50 Blanco FJ, Guitian R, Vazquez-Martul E, *et al.* Osteoarthritis chondrocytes die by apoptosis. A possible pathway for osteoarthritis pathology. *Arthritis Rheum* 1998;**41**:284–9.

51 Hashimoto S, Takahashi K, Amiel D, *et al.* Chondrocyte apoptosis and nitric oxide production during experimentally induced osteoarthritis. *Arthritis Rheum* 1998; **41**:1266–74.

52 Pelletier JP, Mineau F, Ranger P, *et al.* The increased synthesis of inducible nitric oxide inhibits IL-1Ra synthesis by human articular chondrocytes: possible role in osteoarthritic cartilage degradation. *Osteoarthr Cartilage* 1996;**4**:77–84.

53 Zaragoza C, Balbin M, Lopez-Otin C, *et al.* Nitric oxide regulates matrix metalloprotease-13 expression and activity in endothelium. *Kidney Int* 2002;**61**:804–8.

54 Mauviel A, Loyau G, Pujol JP. Effect of unsaponifiable extracts of avocado and soybean (Piascledine) on the collagenolytic action of cultures of human rheumatoid synoviocytes and rabbit articular chondrocytes treated with interleukin-1. *Rev Rhum Mal Osteoartic* 1991;**58**:241–5.

55 Henrotin Y, Labasse A, Jaspar JM, *et al.* Effects of three avocado/soybean unsaponifiable mixtures on metalloproteinases, cytokines and prostaglandin E2 production by human articular chondrocytes. *Clin Rheumatol* 1998;**17**:31–9.

56 Boumediene K, Felisaz N, Bogdanowicz P, *et al.* Avocado/soya unsaponifiables enhance the expression of transforming growth factor beta-1 and beta-2 in cultured articular chondrocytes. *Arthritis Rheum* 1999;**42**:148–56.

57 Omoigui S. The biochemical origin of pain – Proposing a new law of pain: The origin of all pain is inflammation and the inflammatory response. Part 1 of 3 – A unifying law of pain. *Med Hypoth* 2007;**69**:70–82.

58   Kontinnen YT, Kemppinen P, Segerberg M, *et al.* Peripheral and spinal neural mechanisms in arthritis with particular reference to treatment of inflammation and pain. *Arthritis Rheumatol* 1994;**37**:965–82.

59   McDevitt C, Gilbertson E, Muir H. An experimental model of osteoarthritis: early morphological and biochemical changes. *J Bone Joint Surg Br* 1977;**59**:24–38.

60   Moskowitz RW, Goldberg VM. Studies of osteophyte pathogenesis in experimentally induced osteoarthritis. *J Rheumatol* 1987;**14**:311–20.

61   Mine T, Kimura M, Sakka A, *et al.* Innervation of nociceptors in the menisci of the knee joint: an immunohistochemical study. *Arch Orthop Trauma Surg* 2000;**120**:201–4.

62   Fox SM. *Chronic Pain in Small Animal Medicine.* Manson Publishing, London, 2009.

63   Holton L, Reid J, Scott EM, *et al.* Development of a behaviour-based scale to measure acute pain in dogs. *Vet Rec* 2001;**28**:525–31.

64   Wiseman-Orr M, Scott EM, Reid J, *et al.* Validation of a structured questionnaire as an instrument to measure chronic pain in dogs on the basis of effects on health-related quality of life. *Am J Vet Res* 2006;**67**:1826–36.

65   McMillan FD. Quality of life in animals. *JAVMA* 2000;**216**:1904–10.

66   Hielm-Björkman AK, Kuusela E, Markkola A, *et al.* Evaluation of methods for assessment of pain associated with chronic osteoarthritis in dogs. *JAVMA* 2003;**222**:1552–8.

67   Gingerich DA, Strobel JD. Use of client-specific outcome measures to assess treatment effects in geriatric, arthritic dogs: controlled clinical evaluation of a nutraceutical. *Vet Ther* 2003;**4**:56–66.

68   Grieson HA, Summers BA, Lust G. Ultrastructure of the articular cartilage and synovium in the early stages of degenerative joint disease in canine hip joints. *Am J Vet Res* 1982;**43**:1963–71.

69   Boniface RJ, Cain PR, Evans CH. Articular responses to purified cartilage proteoglycans. *Arthritis Rheumatol* 1988;**31**:258–66.

70   Johnston SA. Osteoarthritis: joint anatomy, physiology, and pathobiology. *Vet Clin North Am (SAP)* 1997;**27**:699–723.

71   Burr DB, Radin EL. Trauma as a factor in the initiation of osteoarthritis. In: Brandt KD (ed). *Cartilage Changes in Osteoarthritis.* Indiana University School of Medicine, Indianapolis, 1990, p. 63.

72   Meyers SL, Brandt KD, O'Connor BL, *et al.* Synovitis and osteoarthritic changes in canine articular cartilage after anterior cruciate ligament transection: effect of surgical hemostasis. *Arthritis Rheumatol* 1990;**33**:1406–15.

73   Galloway RH, Lester SJ. Histopathological evaluation of canine stifle joint synovial membrane collected at the time of repair of cranial cruciate ligament rupture. *J Am Anim Hosp Assoc* 1995;**31**:289–94.

74   Bendele AM. Progressive chronic osteoarthritis in femorotibial joints of partial medial meniscectomized guinea pigs. *Vet Pathol* 1987;**24**:444–8.

75   Bendele AM, White SL. Early histopathologic and ultrastructural alterations in femorotibial joints of partial medial meniscectomized guinea pigs. *Vet Pathol* 1987;**24**:436–43.

76   Kamekura S, Hoshi K, Shimoaka T, *et al.* Osteoarthritis development in novel experimental mouse models induced by knee joint instability. *Osteoarthr Cartilage* 2005;**13**:632–41.

77   Bendele AM. Animal models of osteoarthritis. *J Musculoskel Neuron Interact* 2001;**1**:363–76.

78   Brandt KD, Braunstein EM, Visco DM, *et al.* Anterior (cranial) cruciate ligament transection in the dog: a bona fide model of osteoarthritis, not merely of cartilage injury and repair. *J Rheumatol* 1991;**18**:436–46.

79   Oegema TR, Visco D. Animal models of osteoarthritis. In: *Animal Models in Orthopaedic Research.* An YH, Friedman RJ (eds). CRC Press, Boca Raton, 1999, pp. 349–67.

80   Griffiths RJ, Schrier DJ. Advantages and limitations of animals models in the discovery and evaluation of novel disease-modifying osteoarthritis drugs (DMOADs). In: Brandt KD, Doherty M, Lohmander LS (eds). *Osteoarthritis.* Oxford University Press, Oxford, 2003, pp. 411–16.

81   Pritzker KP. Animal models for osteoarthritis: processes, problems, and prospects. *Ann Rheum Dis* 1994;**53**:406–20.

82 Brandt KD, Myers SL, Burr D, *et al.* Osteoarthritic changes in canine articular cartilage, subchondral bone, and synovium fifty-four months after transection of the anterior cruciate ligament. *Arthritis Rheumatol* 1991;**34**:1560–70.

83 Smith GN Jr, Myers SL, Brandt KD, *et al.* Diacerhein treatment reduces the severity of osteoarthritis in the canine cruciate-deficient model of osteoarthritis. *Arthritis Rheumatol* 1999;**42**:545–54.

84 Schawalder P, Gitterle E. Some methods for surgical reconstruction of ruptures of the anterior and posterior crucial ligaments. *Kleintiepraxis* 1989;**34**:323–30.

85 Cox JS, Nye CE, Schaefer WW, *et al.* The degenerative effects of partial and total resection of the medial meniscus in dogs' knees. *Clin Orthop Relat Res* 1975;**109**:178–83.

86 Frost-Christensen LN, Mastbergen SC, Vianen ME, *et al.* Degeneration, inflammation, regeneration, and pain/disability in dogs following destabilization or articular cartilage grooving of the stifle joint. *Osteoarthr Cartilage* 2008;**16**:1327–35.

87 Marijnissen ACA, van Roermund PM, TeKoppele JM, *et al.* The canine 'groove' model, compared with the ACLT model of osteoarthritis. *Osteoarthr Cartilage* 2002;**10**:145–55.

88 Hulse DA, Butler DL, Kay MD, *et al.* Biomechanics of cranial cruciate ligament reconstruction in the dog. 1. In vitro laxity testing. *Vet Surg* 1983;**12**:109–12.

89 Kirby BM. Decision-making in cranial cruciate ligament ruptures. *Vet Clin North Am (SAP)* 1993;**23**:797–819.

90 Lopez MJ, Kunz D, Vanderby R Jr, *et al.* A comparison of joint stability between anterior cruciate intact and deficient knees: a new canine model of anterior cruciate ligament disruption. *J Orthop Res* 2003;**21**:224–30.

91 Vasseur PB. Stifle joint. In: Slatter D (ed). *Textbook of Small Animal Surgery*, edn 3. Vol 2. WB Saunders, Philadelphia, 2003, pp. 2090–133.

92 Slocum B, Slocum TD. Tibial plateau leveling osteotomy for repair of cranial cruciate ligament rupture in the canine. *Vet Clin North Am (SAP)* 1993;**23**:777–95.

93 Montavon PM, Damur DM, Tepic S. Advancement of the tibial tuberosity for the treatment of cranial cruciate deficient canine stifle. *Proceedings of the 1st World Orthopaedic Veterinary Congress.* Munich, Germany, September 2002, p. 152.

94 Lafaver S, Miller NA, Stubbs WP, *et al.* Tibial tuberosity advancement for stabilization of the canine cranial cruciate ligament-deficient stifle joint: surgical technique, early results, and complications in 101 dogs. *Vet Surg* 2007;**36**:573–86.

95 Smith GK, Gregor TP, Rhodes WH, *et al.* Coxofemoral joint laxity from distraction radiography and its contemporaneous and prospective correlation with laxity, subjective score, and evidence of degenerative joint disease from conventional hip-extended radiography in dogs. *Am J Vet Res* 1993;**54**:1021–42.

96 Smith GK, Popovitch CA, Gregor TP, *et al.* Evaluation of risk factors for degenerative joint disease associated with hip dysplasia in dogs. *JAVMA* 1995;**206**:642–7.

97 Smith GK, Mayhew PD, Kapatkin AS, *et al.* Evaluation of risk factors for degenerative joint disease associated with hip dysplasia in German Shepherd Dogs, Golden Retrievers, Labrador Retrievers, and Rottweilers. *JAVMA* 2001;**219**:1719–24.

98 Samoy Y, Van Ryssen B, Gielen I, *et al.* Elbow incongruity in the dog: review of the literature. *Vet Comp Orthop Traumatol* 2006;**19**:1–8.

99 Evans RB, Gordon-Evans WJ, Conzemius MG. Comparison of three methods for the management of fragmented medial coronoid process in the dog. A systematic review and meta-analysis. *Vet Comp Orthop Traumatol* 2008;**21**:106–9.

100 Morgan JP, Wind A, Davidson AP. Osteochondroses, hip dysplasia, elbow dysplasia. In: Morgan JP (ed). *Hereditary Bone and Joint Diseases in the Dog.* Schlütersche GmbH & Co., Hanover, 1999, pp. 41–94.

Chapter 3

Multimodal Management for Canine Osteoarthritis

QUALITY OF EVIDENCE

Quality of evidence is an important consideration when making a therapeutic decision, in that it is the best predictor of consistent clinical outcome. Quality of evidence can be graded from 1 to 4; grades 1 and 2 comprise the highest level of evidence, consisting of systematic reviews (meta-analyses) and well designed, properly randomized, controlled, patient-centered clinical trials (RCCTs). Grade 3 denotes a moderate level of evidence, consisting of well designed, non-RCCTs, epidemiological studies (cohort, case–control), models of disease, and dramatic results in uncontrolled studies. Grade 4 is the lowest level of evidence, encompassing expert opinions, descriptive studies, studies in non-target species, pathophysiologic findings, and in vitro studies (**3.1**). Very few reports have been made reviewing the quality of evidence of treatments for osteoarthritis (OA) in dogs[1,2].

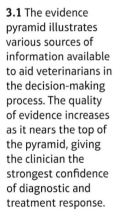

3.1 The evidence pyramid illustrates various sources of information available to aid veterinarians in the decision-making process. The quality of evidence increases as it nears the top of the pyramid, giving the clinician the strongest confidence of diagnostic and treatment response.

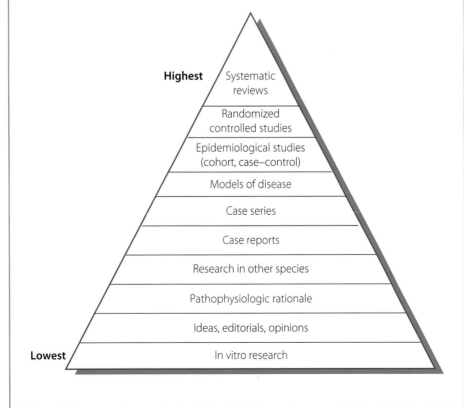

Highest — Systematic reviews

Randomized controlled studies

Epidemiological studies (cohort, case–control)

Models of disease

Case series

Case reports

Research in other species

Pathophysiologic rationale

Ideas, editorials, opinions

Lowest — In vitro research

The multimodal OA management model consists of medical and nonmedical aspects (**3.2**). *Table 3.1* presents evidence for the various therapeutic approaches. The evidence base for each modality of this multimodal management approach is substantial, and impacts on the tenet of determining the minimal effective dose to maximize safety of pharmacologic therapy (specifically, nonsteroidal anti-inflammatory drugs [NSAIDs]).

BACKGROUND

For many years, pain was managed by administration of a single pharmacologic agent (if it was managed at all), and often only when the animal 'proved' to the clinician that it was suffering. Within the past 10–20 years advancements in the understanding of pain physiology, introduction of more efficacious and safer drugs, and the maturation of ethics toward animals have considerably improved the management of pain that our veterinary patients need and deserve.

Following the lead in human medicine, veterinarians have come to appreciate that the network of pain processing involves an incredibly complex and large number of transmitters and receptors, all with different mechanisms, dynamics, and modes of action. From this appreciation comes the conclusion that it is naive to expect effective treatment with a single agent, working by a single mode of action. Multimodal management was initially understood as the administration of a combination of different drugs from different pharmacologic classes such that they act by different, noncompeting modes of action. However, the concept has expanded to include different delivery forms, e.g. oral, systemic, transdermal, transbuccal, intra-articular and epidural; as well as non-pharmacologic modalities such as acupuncture, physical rehabilitation, and regenerative medicine. Intrinsic to the concept is that the drug combination will be synergistic (or at least additive), requiring a reduced amount of each individual drug and, therefore, render less potential for adverse response to each drug within the combination. Selection of drugs within the 'cocktail' would be optimal if they collectively blocked all four of the physiologic pain processes of transduction, transmission, modulation, and perception.

Perioperative multimodal analgesia is widely practiced today in veterinary medicine; however, monotherapy continues to be common practice for managing the chronic pain of OA. NSAIDs are the

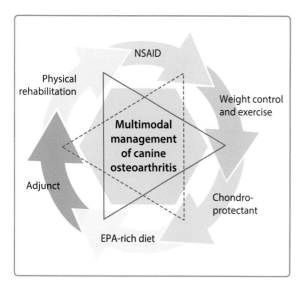

3.2 The multimodal osteoarthritis management 'star' represents two overlapping triangles: medicinal and nonmedicinal. EPA: Eicosapentaenoic acid.

Table 3.1 Evidence for therapeutic approaches to OA

Modality:	Selected references establishing evidence
NSAID	3, 4–6
Chondroprotectant	7–10
Adjuncts	11–13
Weight control/exercise	14–16, 17–19
Eicosapentaenoic acid-rich diet	20–25
Physical rehabilitation	26–29

foundation for treating OA, and are likely to be the foundation for some years to come. Many clinicians manage the elusive pain of OA simply by sequencing different NSAIDs until satisfactory patient results are found or unacceptable adverse reactions are experienced. However, optimal clinical results are most frequently obtained by implementing a multimodal protocol for OA, as has been proved for multimodal perioperative analgesia.

Although contemporary experience precedes published literature, there is a growing evidence base for the multimodal management of OA. This evidence is a collation of clinical expertise, client/patient preferences, available resources, and research evidence, positioned on the evidence pyramid.

MEDICINAL MANAGEMENT

Medicinal management consists of three parts: (1) NSAIDs, (2) chondroprotectants, and (3) adjunct medications/treatments (3.3).

NONSTEROIDAL ANTI-INFLAMMATORY DRUGS

NSAIDs will likely remain the foundation for treating canine OA based on their anti-inflammatory, analgesic, and antipyretic properties. As with all

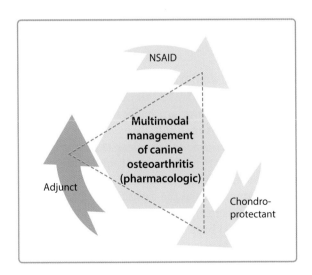

3.3 The medicinal management triangle comprises nonsteroidal anti-inflammatory drugs (NSAIDs), chondroprotectants, and adjunct medications.

drugs, every NSAID has the potential for patient-dependent intolerance. Further, NSAID adverse responses are over-represented by excessive dosing[30,31]. As OA patients age, and possibly experience underlying subclinical renal and/or hepatic compromise, it is imperative that their maintenance NSAID administration be at the minimal effective dose. A multimodal OA treatment protocol is anchored on this tenet of minimal effective dose.

NSAIDs relieve the clinical signs of pain. This is achieved by suppression of prostaglandins (PGs), primarily PGE_2, produced from the substrate arachidonic acid within the prostanoid cascade. PGE_2 plays a number of roles in OA including: 1) lowering the threshold of nociceptor activation; 2) promoting synovitis in the joint lining; 3) enhancing the formation of degradative metalloproteinases (MMPs); and 4) depressing cartilage matrix synthesis by chondrocytes. In contrast, PGs also play positive metabolic roles such as enhancing platelet aggregation (to prevent excessive bleeding), maintaining integrity of the gastrointestinal (GI) tract, and facilitating renal function. Eicosanoid activity is tissue dependent. It is the goal of NSAID management to inhibit PG formation that contributes to the clinical signs and pathways of OA, while sparing PG production associated with beneficial physiologic functions (3.4)[32]. Therefore, maintaining an optimal balance of PG production in the body is the 'NSAID challenge'.

NSAIDs and the COX-1:COX-2 ratio
The IC50 is defined as the concentration of drug (NSAID) needed to inhibit the activity of the enzyme cyclo-oxygenase (COX) by 50%. In keeping with the above rationale, one would like to have a high concentration of NSAID before causing 50% inhibition of COX-1 ('good guy', or beneficial PGs) and a low concentration of NSAID to reach the IC50 for COX-2 ('bad guy', or PGs associated with the pain and pathology of OA):

$$\frac{\text{IC50 of COX-1 (good)} \quad \text{HIGH}}{\text{IC50 of COX-2 (bad)} \quad \text{LOW}}$$

The higher the numerator and lower the denominator, the higher the absolute value. Therefore, a

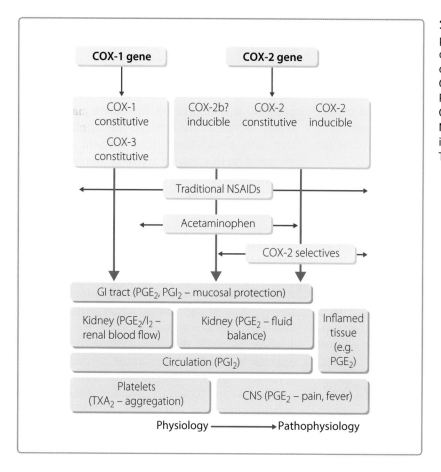

3.4 Cyclo-oxygenase-mediated prostanoids play a variety of physiologic roles, some constitutive, some pathologic[32]. GI: gastrointestinal; PG: prostaglandin; COX: cyclo-oxygenase; NSAID: nonsteroidal anti-inflammatory drug; TX: thromboxane.

greater COX-1/COX-2 ratio suggests (theoretically) the more optimal performing NSAID. With this in mind, pharmaceutical companies began designing NSAIDs for which it takes a low concentration to inhibit COX-2, but a high concentration to inhibit COX-1. Many factors such as species, incubation time, and enzyme source can influence the data obtained from enzyme preparations and *in vitro* testing.

NSAID selection based upon the IC50 ratio can easily be misinterpreted. Firstly, IC50 ratio data are generated *in vitro*. Secondly, the optimal ratio is unknown. It is known that a NSAID can be too COX-2-selective, but the actual magnitude is as yet unknown. What is undisputed is that the optimal NSAID should be COX-1-sparing, appreciating that COX-1 is more responsible for normal constitutive functions such as platelet aggregation, normal renal function, and normal GI function than is

COX-2. This has driven the creation of coxib-class NSAIDs, which are COX-2-selective and (relatively) COX-1-sparing (**3.5**).

Arachidonic acid pathway

In most respects NSAIDs can be characterized as a class, whereas there are molecule-specific characteristics. NSAIDs manifest their mode of action on the arachidonic acid (AA) cascade (**3.6**). It is important to note that the function of many prostanoids is tissue-dependent, e.g. PGs may contribute to pain and inflammation in the arthritic joint, while they enhance normal homeostatic functions of vascularization and bicarbonate and mucus secretion in the GI tract. At one time it was believed that blocking the COX pathway results in a build-up of the substrate AA, which would then lead to increased production of leukotrienes. This has been refuted by some[33], while supported by others[34].

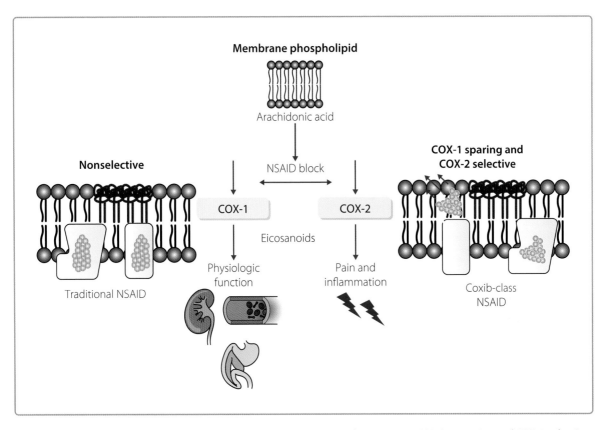

3.5 Summary of the cyclo-oxygenase pathway and nonselective vs. cyclo-oxygenase (COX)-1 sparing and COX-2 selective nonsteroidal anti-inflammatory drugs (NSAIDs). The coxib-class NSAIDs were designed to be too large to fit into the COX-1 receptor site (at label doses), but fit well into the COX-2 receptor site, thereby blocking pathologic COX-2-mediated prostaglandins (PGs), while sparing physiologic COX-1-mediated PGs. This is in contrast to traditional (nonselective) NSAIDs, which fit into both the COX-1 and COX-2 receptors, blocking both COX-1- and COX-2-mediated PGs.

NSAID efficacy and safety

To date, only one study has compared the relative efficacy of multiple contemporary NSAIDs in dogs (n=8)[3]. This study received no commercial funding and used objective assessment (force plate gait analysis). A noteworthy finding in this study was that every dog in the study responded to a NSAID, but not every dog responded to each NSAID (**3.7**).

Currently, several NSAIDs (aspirin, carprofen, cinchophen, deracoxib, etodolac, firocoxib, flunixin, ketoprofen, meloxicam, phenylbutazone, tepoxalin, tolfenamic acid, robenacoxib, mavacoxib, and vedaprofen) have approval for the control of canine perioperative and/or chronic pain in various countries. NSAIDs approved for feline use are far more restricted.

The most common complications documented with NSAID use in the dog are associated with overdosing and the concurrent use with other NSAIDs and/or corticosteroids[35,36]. Because corticosteroids have their mode of action at a location higher in the AA cascade than do NSAIDs, it is redundant to use them concurrently, and doing so markedly increases the severity of adverse reactions[30,37,38]. Data from humans show that the risk of NSAID-induced GI complications is doubled when a NSAID is used concurrently with a corticosteroid[39]. Of adverse reactions reported, as a class of drug, NSAIDs are most commonly associated with adverse reactions to the GI tract (64%), renal system (21%), and liver (14%)[40]. There is no published information relating to similar feline adverse drug events.

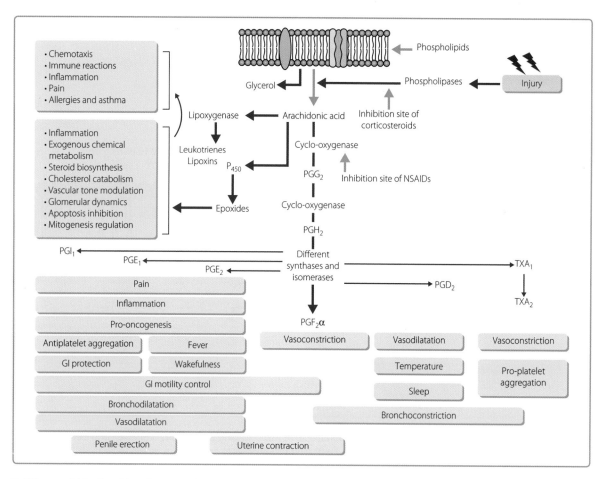

3.6 The arachidonic acid pathway produces a number of eicosanoids that impact on the physiology of joint inflammation. GI: gastrointestinal; PG: prostaglandin; NSAID: nonsteroidal anti-inflammatory drug; TX: thromboxane.

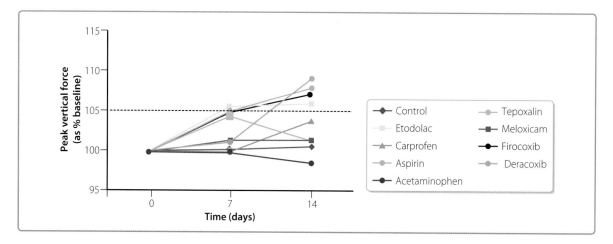

3.7 Relative efficacy of several contemporary nonsteroidal anti-inflammatory drugs (NSAIDs) used in veterinary medicine to treat stifle osteoarthritis. Each dog in the study (n=8) was given each separate NSAID, with a washout period between different NSAIDs. Every dog responded to a NSAID but not every dog responded to each NSAID[3].

NSAIDs and GI function

Development of gastric mucosal hemorrhage, erosion, and ulceration associated with administration of NSAIDs is largely attributed to reduction of PGE synthesis in the gastric mucosa. PGs play a key role in protection of the GI mucosal barrier in: 1) increasing mucus and bicarbonate secretion, 2) enhancing mucosal blood flow, 3) stimulating epithelial cell growth, and 4) suppressing acid secretion.

GI problems associated with NSAIDs can be as benign as regurgitation or as serious as gastric ulceration and perforation. Vomiting has been identified as the most frequent clinical sign associated with gastric perforation[30]. Pet owners should be informed that if their pet experiences vomiting while taking an NSAID, the drug should be stopped and the patient should promptly be examined. This is a conservative approach since dogs are considered a 'vomiting species' and some NSAIDs are associated with more vomiting than others.

NSAIDs and renal function

Through regulation of vascular tone, blood flow, ion and water balance, and renin, PGs are important for normal renal function[41]. In situations of decreased systemic blood pressure or circulating blood volume, PGs assist to regulate and maintain renal blood flow to maintain a mean arterial pressure ranging from 60 to 150 mmHg[42]. Both the COX-1 and the COX-2 isoforms are expressed in the kidneys of dogs, rats, monkeys, and humans where they both play constitutive roles. Therefore, at recommended dosing, no one NSAID is safer than another for renal function in these species. NSAID complications of hypovolemia and hypotension have led to acute renal failure and death in both dogs and cats[43]. Information regarding COX-1 and COX-2 distribution or expression under varying conditions of the feline kidney is unknown.

NSAIDs and hepatic function

Serious liver injury can occur from acetaminophen (paracetamol) overdose in humans and dogs (recommended doses for dogs is 15 mg/kg orally q8–12 hr and toxicity is rarely seen at <100 mg/kg dosing)[44]. Technically, acetaminophen is not a true NSAID since it is considered analgesic but not anti-inflammatory. Acetaminophen toxicity in cats presents primarily as methemoglobinemia and Heinz body anemia, likely from enhanced susceptibility of feline erythrocytes to oxidative injury[45].

Drug-induced hepatopathy (defined as an elevation of liver enzyme values) is a rare, but potentially serious adverse consequence of several drug classes including NSAIDs, volatile anesthetics, antibiotics, antihypertensives, and anticonvulsants. This can occur with all NSAIDs. It is well advised to characterize liver enzymes before and during NSAID administration, especially when an NSAID is being administered long term (*Table 3.2*). However, an increase in liver enzymes is difficult to interpret, as chronic administration of any drug can cause an elevation, and liver enzymes are not a good measure of hepatic function. When liver enzymes

Table 3.2 Approximate plasma half-life of hepatic enzymes in the dog and cat

Enzyme	Dog	Cat
Alanine aminotransferase	40–61 hr	3.5 hr
Aspartate aminotransferase	12 hr	1.5 hr
Glutamate dehydrogenase	18 hr	
Alkaline phosphatase		
Hepatobiliary isoenzyme	66 hr	6 hr
Corticosteroid isoenzyme	74 hr	
Intestinal isoenzyme	6 min	2 min

are elevated and concern for liver function is present, liver function tests should be performed. Mere elevation of liver enzymes may not be cause for discontinuing an NSAID.

NSAID washout time

Currently, there is no evidence-based guidance to address the contemporary question of 'washout' period when changing from one NSAID to a different NSAID. Empirically, it seems appropriate to follow aspirin with a conservative washout of approximately 7 days to allow for platelet regeneration (aspirin irreversibly acetylates platelets), and replacement of the protective protein, aspirin triggered lipoxin. In one study conducted with a limited number of healthy dogs at Colorado State University, there was no significant difference in clinical or clinicopathologic data between dogs that were given an injectable NSAID followed by the same drug in tablet form, and for those dogs given the injectable NSAID followed by a different coxib-class NSAID[46].

Aspirin

Aspirin presents unique risk factors to the canine patient. Aspirin is both topically and systemically toxic (even at low doses of 5–10 mg/kg SID), chondro-destructive, causes irreversible platelet acetylation, and is associated with GI bleeding of as much as 3 ml/day[47,48]. The American Medical Association (AMA) reports that 16,500 people die each year associated with NSAID toxicity[49], yet with an over-representation of patients receiving aspirin. Pet owners often consider aspirin benign because it is available over-the-counter (OTC) and the media suggest it is safe. Even low-dose aspirin has consistently been associated with GI petechiation and hemorrhage. Aspirin does not have a Food and Drug Administration (FDA) license for use in the dog, and the plasma concentrations regarded as being therapeutic are relatively close to the toxic levels[50]. In theory, since aspirin causes GI lesions, it would be inappropriate to progress sequentially from aspirin to a strongly COX-2 selective NSAID (which might restrict the COX-2 necessary for repair following aspirin-induced GI lesions) without an adequate washout period following the aspirin. It is also perilous to use aspirin together with another NSAID or corticosteroid.

In addition to the other effects of PG inhibition on the GI tract, aspirin can cause direct cellular toxicosis, independent of the inhibition of PG synthesis. Aspirin may cause gastric mucosal injury via two mechanisms: 1) direct damage to the gastric epithelial cell, and 2) indirect damage caused by its anti-PG effects[51]. The erosive effects of aspirin on the canine stomach have been known since 1909, when Christoni and Lapressa administered 150–200 mg of aspirin to dogs and noted gastric lesions[52]. Interestingly, the discovery of aspirin's ulcerogenic properties resulted in its use in the study of gastroduodenal ulcer disease in animal models[53,54]. Topical irritation and physical damage to the gastric mucosa barrier may result from a pH-mediated effect of mucosal hydrophobicity and from direct contact between aspirin and gastric epithelium. In the highly acidic gastric lumen, aspirin is mostly non-ionized and lipid-soluble. In this form, it can freely diffuse into mucosal cells where, at neutral pH, aspirin becomes ionized and water-soluble. The water-soluble form cannot penetrate lipid cell membranes and consequently becomes trapped in mucosal cells. The presence of intracellular aspirin causes increased membrane permeability, leading to an influx of hydrogen ions from the gastric lumen or an increased 'back-diffusion' of acid across the gastric mucosal barrier. This increased acid back-diffusion is crucial in initiating and perpetuating mucosal injury. The result is edema, inflammation, hemorrhage, erosions/ulceration, and submucosal capillary damage.

Standard formulations of buffered aspirin do not provide sufficient buffering to neutralize gastric acid or to prevent mucosal injury[55]. Enteric-coated aspirin causes less gastric injury in humans, compared with that from administration of non-buffered or buffered aspirin, but absorption is quite variable, with coated tablets having been observed to pass in the feces[56,57].

NSAIDs and bone healing

Among their many uses, COX inhibitors (NSAIDs) are widely administered for musculoskeletal conditions, including postsurgical orthopedic analgesia. It has been hypothesized that these agents may modulate bone, ligament, or tendon healing by inhibiting PG production. Results from animal models do suggest that NSAIDs and COX-2 inhibitors may have a minimal effect on bone, tendon, and ligament healing, especially at earlier stages, but have no significant impact on the ultimate long-term outcome. In a review on the subject[58], the authors proposed that despite the contribution of PGs to the dynamic process of normal bone healing and pathophysiology, alternative mechanisms may maintain normal bone function in the absence of COX-2 activity. Direct comparison studies suggest that adverse effects of selective COX-2 inhibitors on bone healing are lesser in magnitude than those of nonselective NSAIDs[58].

NSAID compatibility with other agents

NSAIDs are highly protein bound, and may compete with binding of other highly protein bound drugs, particularly in the hypoproteinemic animal, resulting in altered circulating drug concentrations (*Table 3.3*). Fortunately, the number of other highly protein bound drugs is minimal. However, because pet owners tend to be using more and more 'natural' products, some of which can potentially influence the concurrent use of a NSAID, it is well advised to ask owners for a complete listing of everything they are giving their pet orally (*Table 3.4*).

Antiulcer agents

One goal of antiulcer treatment is to lower intragastric acidity to prevent further destruction of the GI tract mucosa. Cimetidine (Tagamet®), a histamine H2-receptor blocker, is commonly used. Cimetidine requires dosing 3–4 times daily; however, it is not effective in preventing NSAID-induced gastric ulceration. Omeprazole (Prilosec®) is a substituted benzimidazole that acts by inhibiting the hydrogen–potassium ATPase (proton pump inhibitor) that is responsible for the production of hydrogen ions in the parietal cell. It is 5–10 times more potent than cimetidine for inhibiting gastric acid secretion and has a long duration of action, requiring once-a-day administration. It may be useful in decreasing gastric hyperacidity, but has minimal effect on ulcer healing. Misoprostol (Cytotec®) is a synthetic PGE_1 analog used to prevent gastric ulceration. It decreases gastric acid secretion, increases bicarbonate and mucus secretion, increases epithelial cell turnover, and increases mucosal blood flow. Both cimetidine and misoprostol require dosing 3–4 times daily and adverse reactions mimic those of gastritis and ulcerations (*Table 3.5*).

Table 3.3 Potential drug interactions with NSAIDs

Drug	May increase the toxicity of	May decrease the efficacy of	Toxicity may be increased by
Classical NSAIDs (clinically significant COX-1 inhibition)	Warfarin, methotrexate, valproic acid, midazolam, furosemide, spironolactone, sulfonylureas, heparin	Furosemide, thiazide, ACE inhibitors, β-blockers	Aminoglycosides, furosemide, cyclosporine (renal), glucocorticoids (GI), heparin, gingko, garlic, ginger, ginseng (hemorrhage)
Coxibs and relatively COX-2 selective agents	Warfarin, methotrexate, valproic acid, midazolam, furosemide, spironolactone, sulfonylureas	Furosemide, thiazides, ACE inhibitors, β-blockers	Aminoglycosides, furosemide, cyclosporine (renal), glucocorticoids (GI)
Phenylbutazone, acetaminophen	Warfarin, sulfonylureas		Phenobarbital, alcohol, rifampin, metoclopramide

Trepanier LA. Potential interactions between nonsteroidal anti-inflammatory drugs and other drugs. *J Vet Emergency and Critical Care* 2005;**15**(4):248–53[59].

Table 3.4 Potential interactions of drugs with herbs

Herb	Interacting drugs	Results
St. John's wort	Cyclosporine, fexofenadine, midazolam, digoxin, tacrolimus, amitriptyline, warfarin, theophylline	Decreased plasma drug concentrations
Gingko	Warfarin Heparin **NSAIDs** Omeprazole	Bleeding Decreased plasma concentrations
Ginseng	Warfarin Heparin **NSAIDs** Opioids	Bleeding Falsely elevated serum digoxin levels (laboratory test interaction with ginseng) Decreased analgesic effect (laboratory test interaction with ginseng)
Garlic Chamomile Ginger	Warfarin Heparin **NSAIDs**	Bleeding
Devil's claw	**NSAIDs**	Decreases gastric pH

Goodman L, Trepanier L. Potential drug interactions with dietary supplements. *Compendium* (*SAP*) October 2005, 780–789[60].

Table 3.5 'Protective' pharmacologic agents for the gastrointestinal tract

Group	Generic name	Brand name	Dose
Proton pump inhibitors (PPI)	Omeprazole Lansoprazole Rabeprazole Pantoprazole Esomeprazole	Prilosec PrevAcid AcipHex Protonix Nexium	Canine: 0.7 mg/kg, PO
Prostaglandin analog	Misoprostol	Cytotec	Canine: 2–5 µg/kg, tid, PO
H2-receptor blockers	Cimetidine	Tagamet	Canine/feline: 10 mg/kg, tid, PO, IV, IM Feline: 3.5 mg/kg, bid, PO or 2.5 mg/kg, bid, IV
	Ranitidine	Zantac	Canine: 2 mg/kg, tid, PO, IV
	Famotidine	Pepcid	Canine/feline: 0.5 mg/kg, sid, PO, IV, IM, SQ or 0.25 mg/kg, bid, PO, IV, IM, SQ
	Nizatidine	Axid	Canine: 2.5–5 mg/kg, sid, PO
Mucosal sealant	Sucralfate	Carafate	Canine: 0.5–1 g, tid-bid, PO Feline: 0.25 g, tid-bid, PO

Cats and NSAIDs

There are approximately 82 million cats in the USA[61] and approximately 10 million in the UK[62]. Radiographically, degenerative joint disease is apparently detectable in as high as 90% of cats over 12 years of age[63]. Efficacy of NSAIDs for relief of chronic pain in the cat is difficult to demonstrate, but empirically embraced. Objective measurement of lameness severity in cats is quite difficult, as cats do not comply with force plate protocols. However, pressure mats have been used to reveal the distribution of pressures associated with paw contact[64], so that pressures on each digital pad and on the metacarpal pad could be measured quantitatively following onychectomies. Use of the pressure mat to evaluate lameness in cats will likely see further development. The use of acceleration-based activity monitors may also allow for future objective measurement of improved mobility following treatment for osteoarthritic conditions in the cat[65]. Probable reasons for the relative void of evidence base for NSAIDs in cats include:

- Assumption by pharmaceutical manufacturers that the market for cat analgesics is not financially rewarding.
- Difficulty of identifying pain in cats, and therefore indications for administration.
- Scarcity of information about NSAIDs in cats.
- Potential risk of NSAID toxicity in cats.

Salicylate toxicity in cats is well established. Cats present a unique susceptibility for NSAID toxicity because of slow clearance and dose-dependent elimination. Cats have a low capacity for hepatic glucuronidation of NSAIDs[66], which is the major mechanism of metabolism and excretion for this class of drugs. Acetaminophen toxicity in cats results in methemoglobinemia, liver failure, and death. Cats are particularly susceptible to acetaminophen toxicity due, in part, to defective conjugation of the drug and conversion to a reactive electrolytic metabolite. Because of its delivery form as an elixir, meloxicam is sometimes used preferentially in small dogs and cats. However, only carprofen, meloxicam, and robenacoxib injectables are approved for use in the cat (country dependent) and manufacturers stress limited dosing only. There are sparse data to support the safe chronic use of NSAIDs in cats[67].

The manufacturer of meloxicam has recommended reducing the original approval dose from 0.2 to 0.1 mg/kg because of some initial GI problems. This suggests particular attention be given to accurate dosing of small dogs and cats. As with all NSAIDs in dogs or cats, potentially causal gastric ulcerations have been observed.

Enhancing responsible NSAID use

Every pet owner who is discharged with medication, including NSAIDs, should have the following questions addressed:

1. What is the medication supposed to do?
2. What are the proper dose and dosing interval?
3. What potential adverse response(s) are possible?
4. What should I do if I observe an adverse response?

Both verbal and written instructions should be given. Preadministrative urinalysis and blood chemistries are well advised prior to dispensing NSAIDs for two primary reasons. Firstly, the pet may be a poor candidate for any NSAID, i.e. it may be azotemic or have decreased liver function. These physiologic compromises may not preclude the use of NSAIDs, but such a determination must be carefully considered and justified. Secondly, a baseline status should be established for subsequent comparison, should the patient show clinical signs suggestive of drug intolerance. For the patient on a long-term NSAID protocol, the frequency of laboratory profiling should be determined by clinical signs and age. Minimal effective dose should always be the therapeutic objective, and routine examinations of the animal constitute the practice of good medicine. Since alanine aminotransferase (ALT) is more specific than serum alkaline phosphatase (SAP) as a blood chemistry for liver status, an elevation 3–4 times greater than normal laboratory values should prompt a subsequent liver function test. Because the kidney expresses both COX isozymes constitutively, no one NSAID can be presumed safer than another for renal function, and any patient that is hypotensive or insufficiently hydrated is at risk for adverse events secondary to NSAID administration.

NSAIDs play a major role in a perioperative protocol for healthy animals, due to their features as anti-inflammatories, analgesics, and antipyretics. NSAID inclusion helps prevent CNS 'wind up', and there is synergism with opioids[68]. Surgery cannot be performed without resultant iatrogenic inflammation, and the best time to administer the anti-inflammatory drug is pre-emptively, before the surgery. It is imperative that surgical patients be sufficiently hydrated if NSAIDs are used perioperatively. Under the influence of gaseous anesthesia, renal tissue may suffer from under-perfusion, at which point PGs are recruited to assist with this perfusion; if the patient is under the influence of an anti-PG (NSAID), the patient may be at risk for acute renal failure. In human medicine, some suggest that concerns about postoperative renal impairment should not impact on NSAID administration in adults with normal preoperative renal function[69].

Improving safety

The following guidelines may reduce the risk of NSAID adverse drug events (ADEs):

- Proper dosing.
- Administer minimal effective dose.
- Dispense in approved packaging together with owner information sheets.
- Avoid concurrent use of multiple NSAIDs and NSAIDs with corticosteroids.
- Do not use with aspirin.
- Provide pet owners with both oral and written instructions for responsible NSAID use.
- Conduct appropriate patient chemistry/urine profiling.
- Conduct routine check ups and chemistry profiles for patients on chronic NSAID regimens. Do not fill NSAID prescriptions without conducting patient examinations.
- Caution pet owners regarding supplementation with OTC NSAIDs.
- Administer GI protectants for high at-risk patients on NSAIDs.
- Avoid NSAID administration in puppies and pregnant animals.
- NSAIDs may decrease the action of angiotensin-converting enzyme (ACE) inhibitors and furosemide, a consideration for patients being treated for cardiovascular disease.
- Geriatric animals are more likely to be treated with NSAIDs and other medications on a chronic schedule, therefore their 'polypharmacy' protocols and potentially compromised drug clearance should be considered.
- Provide sufficient hydration to surgery patients administered NSAIDs.
- Report ADEs to the product manufacturer.

Contemporary NSAIDs for use in companion animals and pharmacokinetics of NSAIDs are presented in *Table 3.6* and *Table 3.7*, respectively.

PROSTAGLANDIN E$_2$ RECEPTOR EP4: PIPRANT DRUG CLASS

PGE$_2$ is the principal proinflammatory prostanoid of the AA cascade and contributes, in particular, to one of the key features of inflammation, pain hypersensitivity. At the site of inflammation, PGE$_2$ sensitizes peripheral nociceptors through activation of EP receptors present on the peripheral terminals of these high-threshold sensory neurons, reducing threshold and increasing responsiveness – the phenomenon of peripheral sensitization[70]. PGE$_2$ is also produced in the spinal cord after tissue injury where it contributes to central sensitization, an increase in excitability of spinal dorsal horn neurons that produces pain hypersensitivity[71].

PGE$_2$ exerts its cellular effects through four different G-protein-coupled EP receptors (EP1, EP2, EP3, and EP4). Studies have shown that EP4 is a major receptor in mediating pain associated with both rheumatoid arthritis and OA, and further that an EP4 antagonist is as effective as a COX-2 inhibitor in suppressing joint inflammation – pin pointing EP4 as the principal EP receptor for PGE2[72,73]. In dorsal root ganglion cultures pretreated with EP3C and EP4 antagonists, PGE$_2$-augmented release of substance P and calcitonin gene-related peptide is abolished[74]. Unlike COX-2 inhibitors, EP4 antagonists do not suppress PGI$_2$, which possesses potent vasodilatory and antithrombic activities, and may be cardioprotective (in humans)[75]. Selective EP4 antagonists are different from NSAIDS and COX-2 inhibitors, as they do not inhibit the AA cascade. Since they directly block the action of PGE$_2$, it is expected that they will not exhibit the same side effects as NSAIDs and COX-2 inhibitors.

Table 3.6 Contemporary NSAIDs labeled for companion animal use (labeled use may vary by country)

Active agent	Deracoxib	Carprofen	Firocoxib	Mavacoxib
Company	Novartis/Elanco	Pfizer/Zoetis	Merial	Pfizer/Zoetis
Formulation	25 mg, 75 mg, 100 mg scored chewable tablets	Caplets/chewable tablets: 25, 75, 100 mg scored caplets or scored chewable tablets SQ injectable: 50 mg carprofen/ml	Chewable tablets containing 57 or 227 mg	6, 20, 30, 75 and 95 mg chewable, triangular shaped tablets
Dosage	For the control of pain and inflammation associated with orthopedic surgery in dogs: 3–4 mg/kg; up to 7 days. Give prior to surgery for postoperative pain. For the control of pain and inflammation associated with OA in dogs: 1–2 mg/kg daily	Oral and injectable: 2 mg/lb (4.4 mg/kg) daily: may be administered once daily or divided as 1 mg/lb (2.2 mg/kg) twice daily. For postoperative pain, administer 2 hr before the procedure	5 mg/kg oral once daily. Tablets are scored and dosage should be calculated in ½ tablet increments	MONTHLY TREATMENT: initial dose (2 mg/kg), with food repeated 14 days later, and then monthly dosing for up to a maximum of 7 consecutive doses
Indications	For the control of pain and inflammation associated with orthopedic surgery in dogs weighing >4 lb (1.8 kg). For the control of pain and inflammation associated with OA	For the relief of pain and inflammation associated with OA in dogs and the control of postoperative pain in soft tissue and orthopedic surgeries in dogs	For the control of pain and inflammation associated with OA in dogs	For the treatment of pain and inflammation in dogs aged 12 months or more associated with degenerative joint disease in dogs in cases where continuous treatment exceeding one month is indicated
Mechanism of action	A coxib class drug that uniquely targets COX-2 while sparing COX-1	Inhibition of COX enzyme; *in vitro* selective against COX-2	Inhibition of COX activity; *in vitro* studies show it to be highly selective for COX-2 in canine blood	A coxib-class NSAID that targets COX-2, while sparing COX-1
Maximum concentration (C_{max})	At 2 hr	Oral: C_{max} of 16.9 μg/ml at 0.5–3 hr Injectable: C_{max} of 8.0 μg/ml at 1.5–8 hr		Increases with exposure (day 1–7)
Half-life ($T_{1/2}$)	3 hr	8 hr in dog	7.8 hr	16.6 days (range: 7.9–38.8)

(Table 3.6 continued on next page)

Table 3.6 *continued*

Active agent	Deracoxib	Carprofen	Firocoxib	Mavacoxib
Company	Novartis/Elanco	Pfizer/Zoetis	Merial	Pfizer/Zoetis
Metabolism and excretion	Metabolism primarily liver; excretion in feces is 75%, urine excretion is 20%	Liver biotransformation: 70–80% in feces and 10–20% in urine. Some enterohepatic recirculation	Primarily hepatic metabolism and fecal excretion	Liver metabolism and excreted primarily in feces.
Side-effects within licensing studies. Serious adverse reactions with this drug class can occur without warning and (rarely) result in death	Vomiting, incisional lesions	Black or tarry stools, hypoalbuminemia, dermatologic changes, increased liver enzyme levels, idiosyncratic hepatotoxicosis	Vomiting, diarrhea, decreased appetite. (Use of this product at doses above the recommended 5 mg/kg in puppies <7 months of age has been associated with serious ADEs, including death)	Most common side-effects are loss of appetite, diarrhea and vomiting
Packaging	30 count, 90 count	14, 60, 150 count 20 ml bottle of injectable	10 and 30 count blister packs, 60 count bottles	Carton boxes each contain one blister. Each blister contains two tablets
Marketing	By prescription only	By prescription only	By prescription only	By prescription only
Protein binding	>90%	>99%	>96%	Approximately 98%
Bio-availability	>90%	>90%	Nearly 100%	Approximately 50% when fasted; approximately 90% in fed conditions
Concurrent use treatments, with statement	Concomitant use with any other anti-inflammatory drugs, such as other NSAIDs and corticosteroids, should be avoided or closely monitored Concomitant corticosteroids, anesthetic/analgesic products and tranquilizers could potentially bias efficacy			
Pre-Rx advisement	Thorough history and physical exam; appropriate laboratory tests Dogs with hepatic disorders should not be treated			
Miscellaneous			*In vitro*: showed more COX-2 inhibition than COX-1	May undergo enterohepatic recycling
Active agent	**Meloxicam**	**Etodolac**	**Tepoxalin**	**Robenacoxib**
Company	Boehringer-Ingelheim	Fort Dodge	Schering-Plough	Novartis/Elanco
Formulation	Liquid suspension: to be squirted on food Injectable: 5 mg/ml, SQ or IV	150 mg, 300 mg scored tablets	Rapidly disintegrating tablets of 30, 50, 100, or 200 mg	Dog: 5, 10, 20, 40 mg tablet Cat: 6 mg tablet with NA on one side and AK on the other side. 20 mg/ml SQ injection for cats.

Active agent	Meloxicam	Etodolac	Tepoxalin	Robenacoxib
Company	Boehringer-Ingelheim	Fort Dodge	Schering-Plough	Novartis/Elanco
Dosage	0.2 mg/kg injectable once or oral once: followed by 0.1 mg/kg oral suspension daily. Cats: 0.3 mg/kg presurgical one-time dose (contraindicated to follow in cats with another NSAID or additional doses of meloxicam)	10–15 mg/kg once daily (4.5– 6.8 mg/lb). Adjust dose until a satisfactory clinical response is obtained, i.e. reduce to minimum effective dose	10 mg/kg orally or 20 mg/kg on the initial day of treatment, followed by a daily maintenance dose of 10 mg/kg	Dog: 1 mg/kg sid Cat: 1 mg/kg sid for maximum of 6 days. Injection: 2 mg/kg subcutaneously once daily for a maximum of 3 days.
Indications	Control of pain and inflammation associated with OA in dogs; postoperative pain and inflammation associated with orthopedic surgery, ovariohysterectomy and castration in cats when administered prior to surgery	For the management of pain and inflammation associated with OA in dogs	For the control of postoperative pain and inflammation associated with soft tissue surgery as well as chronic osteoarthritis in dogs. etc.	For the treatment of pain and inflammation associated with chronic osteoarthritis in dogs. For the treatment of acute pain and inflammation associated with musculo-skeletal disorders in cats
Mechanism of action	MOA not on label; oxicam class NSAID	Inhibition of COX activity; inhibits macrophage chemotaxis	COX and LOX inhibitor: 'dual pathway inhibitor of AA metabolism'	A coxib-class NSAID that targets COX-2, while sparing COX-1
Maximum concentration (Cmax)	Dogs: 2.5 hr (inj) and 7.5 hr (oral) Cats: 1.5 hr postinjection	1.08–1.6 hr	2.3±1.4 hr	Dog: <1 hour Cat: 1 hour
Half-life ($T_{1/2}$)	Dogs: 24 hr Cats: 15 hr postinjection	7.6–12 hr	2.0±1.2 hr; converts to active metabolite with long $T_{1/2}$	Dog: 1.2 hours Cat: 1.7 hours
Metabolism and excretion	Not on label	Primarily hepatic metabolism and fecal excretion; enterohepatic recirculation	Primarily hepatic with excretion through feces 99%, minor urine	Mainly metabolized in the liver of both cat and dog, similar to its human analogue, lumiracoxib – primarily via oxidation and hydroxylation. Direct glucuronic acid conjugation is relatively minor

(Table 3.6 continued on next page)

Table 3.6 *continued*

Active agent	Meloxicam	Etodolac	Tepoxalin	Robenacoxib
Company	Boehringer-Ingelheim	Fort Dodge	Schering-Plough	Novartis/Elanco
Side-effects within licensing studies. Serious adverse reactions with this drug class can occur-without warning and (rarely) result in death	Vomiting, soft stools, diarrhea, inappetance, epiphora, auto-immune hemolytic anemia, thrombocytopenia, polyarthritis, pyoderma	Weight loss, fecal abnormalities, hypoproteinemia, small-intestine erosions	Vomiting, diarrhea, gastric lesions, decrease in total protein, albumin and calcium, death	Dogs: GI adverse events reported very commonly, recovering with treatment. Cats: mild and transient diarrhea, soft feces or vomiting commonly reported
Packaging	Oral: 1.5 mg/ml: 10, 32 and 100 ml dropper bottles Inj: 5 mg/ml in a 10 ml vial	7, 30, and 90 count	Boxes containing 10 foil blisters each	Dogs: Boxes containing 1,2, 4 or 10 blisters, 7 tablets each. Cats: Boxes containing 1,2,5 or 10 blisters, 6 tablets each. 20 ml vial.
Marketing	By prescription only	By prescription only	By prescription only	By prescription only
Protein binding	>99%	>99%	>98%	>99%
Bio-availability Concurrent use statement	Nearly 100% Concurrent use with potentially nephro-toxic drugs should be carefully approached. Concomitant use with other anti-inflammatory drugs, such as NSAIDs and corticosteroids, should be avoided or closely monitored	Nearly 100% Concomitant use with any other anti-inflammatory drugs, such as other NSAIDs and cortico-steroids, should be avoided or closely monitored	Do not use concomitantly with corticosteroids or other NSAIDs	Dog: 62% with food; 84% without food. Cat: 49% without food
Pre-Rx advisement	Thorough history and physical exam; appropriate laboratory tests		Geriatric examination; appropriate laboratory tests	Safety not established in cats <2.5 kg or <4 months old
Miscellaneous	Not evaluated for IM injection	*In vitro*: showed more COX-2 inhibition than COX-1	Give with a meal to enhance absorption	Inadequate response to treatment was seen in 10-15% of dogs. In cats: COX-1/COX-2 ratio = 197.5

Table 3.7 Half-life at different doses of various NSAIDs in dogs and cats. As noted, the half-life may change, dependent upon dose and/or route of administration. Numbers within the reference column refer to references citing the respective findings.

NSAID	Half-life (hr)	Dose/route	Reference	Species difference	Clearance/ mechanism
Acetaminophen					Glucuronidation and sulfation
Dog	1.2	100 mg/kg PO	68		
		200 mg/kg PO	68		
Cat				Do not use	
Aspirin					Glucuronidation and glycination
Dog	7.5–12	*25 mg/kg PO*	69	Cat > dog	
Cat	22	*20 mg/kg IV*	70		
	37.6	*IV?*	71		
Carprofen				Cat > dog	Glucuronidation and oxidation
Dog	5	25 mg PO	72		
	8.6	25 mg bid PO 7 d	72		
	7	25 mg SC	72		
	8.3	25 mg bid SC 7 d	72		
Cat	20	4 mg/kg IV	70		
	19	4 mg/kg SC, IV	73		
Deracoxib					
Dog	8	1–2 mg/kg PO	74		
Cat				Do not use	
Flunixin				Cat < dog	Glucuronidation and active transport
Dog	3.7	1.1 mg/kg IV	75		
Cat	1–1.5	1 mg/kg PO, IV	76		
	6.6	2 mg/kg PO	77		
Ketoprofen				Cat = dog	Glucuronidation and thioesterification
Dog	1.6 for S-k	*1 mg/kg PO racemic*	78		
Cat	1.5 for S-k	2 mg/kg IV racemic	79		
	0.6 for R-k	2 mg/kg IV racemic	79		
	0.9 for S-k	1 mg/kg PO racemic	79		
	0.6 for R-k	1 mg/kg PO racemic	79		
	0.5 for S-k	1 mg/kg IV S-k	79		
	0.5 for R-k	1 mg/kg IV R-k	79		

(Table 3.7 continued on next page)

Table 3.7 *continued*

NSAID	Half-life (hr)	Dose/route	Reference	Species difference	Clearance/ mechanism
Mavacoxib				Bile excretion	
Dog	13.8–39 days	2 mg/kg PO q14 days for 2 doses; then q30 days (6.5 mo max dosing)	Label		
Cat				Do not use	
Meloxicam				Cat > dog	Oxidation
Dog	12	0.2 mg/kg PO	80		
	24	0.2 mg/kg PO, SC, IV	80		
Cat	15	0.3 mg/kg SC	Label		
Piroxicam				Cat < dog	Oxidation
Dog	40	*0.3 mg/kg PO, IV*	81		
Cat	12	*0.3 mg/kg PO, IV*	82		
Robenacoxib					65–70% biliary clearance
Dog	1.2	1–2 mg/kg PO	83		
Cat	1.1	1–2.4 mg/kg PO (6 d max dosing)	84		
Tepoxalin					
Dog	1.6	20 mg/kg PO initial dose, then 10 mg/kg	Label		
Cat				Do not use	

NOTE: These doses/route of administration are not recommended doses. **See specific drug labels for recommended dosing.**

The World Health Organization (WHO) has recently (in 2013) recognized a new drug class (**3.8**) for agents targeting the EP receptors with the suffix '—piprant', of which grapiprant was approved in March 2016 for the control of osteoarthritic pain and inflammation in dogs.

DISEASE MODIFYING OSTEOARTHRITIC AGENTS

Polysulfated glycosaminoglycan
A polysulfated glycosaminoglycan (PSGAG) is available as a disease modifying osteoarthritic drug (Adequan®), as is a hyaluronic acid product (Legend™). Other products (e.g. Chondroprotec™ and IChON®), often considered nutraceuticals, are not drugs that have been through the approval process. Such agents are nutritional supplements, while others are licensed as topical wound devices, rather than drugs.

The PSGAG is characterized as a 'disease modifying osteoarthritic drug' which has met the rigors of FDA registration. Experiments conducted *in vitro* have shown PSGAG to inhibit certain catabolic enzymes which have increased activity in inflamed joints, and to enhance the activity of some anabolic

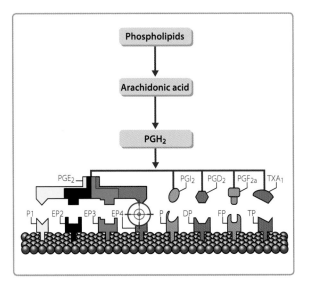

3.8 EP4 is the target receptor site for the new class of piprant drugs. PG: prostaglandin; TX: thromboxane.

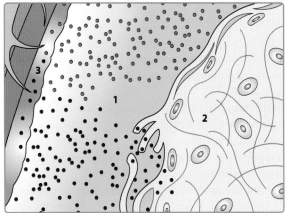

3.9 Cyclic catabolism of osteoarthritis. Inflammatory cytokines (1) (matrix metalloproteinases: MMPs) are released from the diseased cartilage (2) into the synovial fluid, where they contact synoviocytes of the joint capsule lining (intima) (3). These synoviocytes then act like macrophages, releasing additional inflammatory mediators into the synovial fluid, which find their way back into the cartilage matrix with loading/unloading of the mobilized joint.

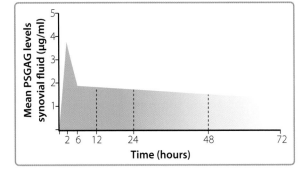

3.10 Polysulfated glycosaminoglycan (PSGAG) Adequan Canine® promptly enters the synovial fluid and lingers for several days.

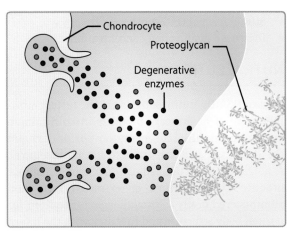

3.11 Polysulfated glycosaminoglycan (PSGAG) mode of action. The traumatized/diseased chondrocyte releases degenerative enzymes (dark circles) which subsequently degrade the cartilage matrix proteoglycans (pink). The PSGAG (green haze) prevents this degradative activity.

enzymes[76]. PSGAG has been shown to significantly inhibit serine proteinases, which play a role in the interleukin (IL)-1-mediated degradation of cartilage proteoglycans and collagen[77]. PSGAG has further been reported to inhibit some catabolic enzymes such as elastase, stromelysin, MMPs, cathepsin G and B1, and hyaluronidases, which degrade collagen, proteoglycans, and hyaluronic acid (**3.9**)[78,79]. It is also reported to inhibit PGE synthesis[80]. PSGAG has shown a specific potentiating effect on hyaluronic acid synthesis by synovial membrane cells *in vitro*[81]. Within 2 hours of administration, the PSGAG enters cartilage (**3.10**) where it reduces proteoglycan degradation, inhibits synthesis and activity of degradative enzymes, stimulates GAG synthesis, and increases hyaluronan concentrations (**3.11**).

Clinical data from Millis *et al.* (unpublished, 2005) showed that comfortable angle of extension and lameness scores were both improved following administration of Adequan PSGAG at both 4 and 8 weeks following cranial cruciate ligament transection (CCLT), while the concentration of neutral MMP was reduced relative to transected controls. In an era when evidence-based treatment is being emphasized, the separation between patient response to FDA-approved drugs and unlicensed agents is widening.

The licensed PSGAG Adequan is most appropriately administered in the early stages of OA, since once hyaline cartilage is lost, it is lost forever! The strategy in administering this chondroprotective early is to delay medically aggressive treatment as long as possible during the progression of OA. PSGAG activity thus offers:

- Reduction in proteoglycan degradation.
- Inhibition of synthesis and activity of:
  - aggrecanases.
  - MMPs.
  - nitric oxide.
  - PGE$_2$.
- Stimulation of GAG synthesis.
- Increased hyaluronan concentrations.

NUTRACEUTICALS

Next to NSAIDs, nutraceuticals are the fastest growing group of health care products in both human and animal health. Yet, many do not understand the definition and constraints of a nutraceutical. A nutraceutical is defined as a nondrug substance produced in a purified or extracted form and administered orally to provide agents required for normal body structure and function, with the intent of improving health and wellbeing. Note that there is no mention of 'scientifically proven'; however, several studies suggest nutraceutical efficacy may be 'not inferior' to approved NSAIDs. Regardless, nutraceuticals are not closely regulated by the FDA and cannot have label claims for treating, curing or mitigating a disease. In contrast, drugs such as PSGAGs are FDA-regulated. Together, chondroprotectants (both injectables and oral nutraceuticals) are considered disease modifying osteoarthritic agents (DMOAAs), whereas nutraceuticals are not considered disease modifying osteoarthritic drugs (DMOADs). More than 30 nutraceutical products have been listed as potentially active in OA (*Table 3.8*)[82].

NSAIDs have become the default 'standard' for comparing OA 'medicinal' efficacy (**3.12**), because agents such as nutraceuticals are not allowed to make therapeutic claims.

Omega-3 fatty acids

Essential fatty acids are a group of polyunsaturated fatty acids that contain both omega-6 fatty acid AA and the omega-3 fatty acids eicosapentaenoic acid (EPA) and docosahexaenoic acid (DHA). Arachidonic acid is incorporated into cell membranes, which are broken down in osteoarthritic joints. When metabolized, it yields inflammatory components, such as PGs, leukotrienes, and thromboxanes.

Table 3.8 Nutraceuticals used in OA

Ascorbic acid	Hyaluronic acid
Avocado/soybean unsaponifiables	Hydrolysate collagen
Boswellia serrata	Methylsulfonylmethane
Bromelain	Milk and hyperimmune milk
Cat's claw	n3-polyunsaturated fatty acids
Chondroitin sulfate	Phycocyanin
Cetyl myristoleic oil	*Ribes nigrum*
Collagen hydrolysate	*Rosa canina*
Curcumin	S-adenosylmethionine (SAMe)
Chitosan	Selenium
Devil's claw	Strontium
Flavonoids	Silicium
Glucosamine SO$_4$/Acetyl/HCl	Turmeric
Green lip mussel	Vitamin D
Ginger	Vitamin E
	Willow bark

Many anti-inflammatory drugs used to manage OA inhibit the conversion of AA into these components. The omega-3 fatty acids are able to compete with and replace omega-6 fatty acids in cell membranes, thus reducing the inflammatory response. Several studies have shown that omega-3 fatty acids have anti-inflammatory properties and therapeutic effects to the cartilage[83–91]. Furthermore, recent studies in dogs with OA have shown that dietary supplementation with omega-3 fatty acids can improve owner perception of comfort and function, improve weight bearing in the affected limb, and decrease the need for NSAIDs[92–95]. In short, when the omega-3 fatty acid replaces AA in cell membranes, the inflammatory cascade is down-regulated. The optimal dietary n6:n3 ratio is unresolved; however, ~5:1 is commonly advised.

Glucosamine/chondroitin

About 21 million Americans have OA[96]. NSAIDs are the foundation for treating OA, but ongoing controversy over conventional medications and their potential for adverse side affects has created fertile soil for the growth of alternative arthritis remedies, particularly glucosamine and chondroitin. First popularized by the 1997 best-seller *The Arthritis Cure*, by Dr. Jason Theodosakis, these supplements racked up combined sales of $640 million in 2000, according to the *Nutrition Business Journal* (*NBJ*). Estimated sales of human-use glucosamine and chondroitin sulfate in 2004 approached $730 million. It would appear that popularity of these supplements in the human sector is driving veterinary use. The world market for pet nutraceuticals was worth $960 million in 2004. About 60% of this was given to dogs, 25% to cats

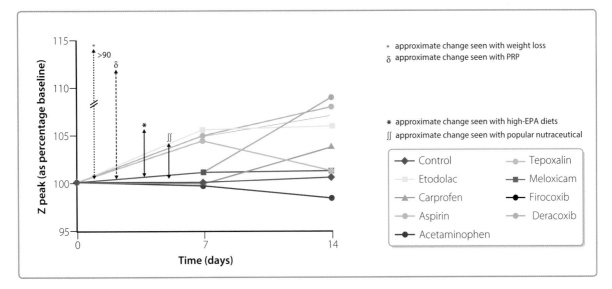

3.12 Nonsteroidal anti-inflammatory drugs (NSAIDs) have become the default 'standard' for comparing osteoathritis 'medicinal' efficacy, because agents such as nutraceuticals are not allowed to make therapeutic claims. Appreciating the inherent issues of comparing data from different studies, response from different treatment modalities, including nutraceuticals, is made to different NSAIDs as assessed by force plate gait analysis. EPA: eicosapentaenoic acid: PRP: platelet-rich plasma.

Millis DL. A multimodal approach to treating osteoarthritis. 2006 Western Veterinary Conference Symposium Proceedings (comparing relative efficacy of various NSAIDs by force plate gait analysis in cruciate deficient dogs)

* Clinician's Update™, Supplement to NAVC Clinician's Brief®. April 2005

δ Fahle MA, *et al.* A randomized controlled trial of the efficacy of autologous platelet therapy for the treatment of osteoarthritis in dogs. *JAVMA* Vol 243, No. 9 2013; 1291–1297

* Effects of feeding omega-3 fatty acids on force plate gait analysis in dogs with osteoarthritis, 3-month feeding study, 2003. Hill's clinical evidence report. Technical information services 2005.

ʃʃ Millis DL. Dasuquin's efficacy may be similar to that of NSAIDs in dogs. Joint Health: a roundtable discussion. (Nutramax Laboratories Inc.) Veterinary Medicine 2010:p.10

and 10% to horses[97]. In 2008, the global nutraceutical supplement market (human and veterinary) was approximately $40 billion. Pet supplements and nutraceuticals are expected to reach sales of $1.6 billion in the year 2015, up 27% from the year 2010. According to *NBJ*, Boulder, CO, natural and organic pet foods, pet supplements, and other natural and organic pet supplies grew 5.2% in 2010 to reach $3.2 billion, with the animal supplement category alone adding $80 million in new sales dollars to reach $1.6 billion. Joint health products for pets account for nearly half of the market, followed by vitamins, minerals, amino acids, and antioxidants with 20%.

A meta-analysis of studies evaluating the efficacy of these supplements for OA suggested potential benefit from these agents, but as is often the case with nutraceuticals, questions were raised about the scientific quality of the studies[98]. Therefore, the Glucosamine/chondroitin Arthritis Intervention Trial (GAIT), a 24-week, randomized, double-blind, placebo- and celecoxib-controlled, multicenter, $14 million trial was sponsored by the National Institutes of Health (NIH), to evaluate rigorously the efficacy and safety of glucosamine, chondroitin sulfate, and the two in combination in the treatment of pain due to human OA of the knee. The primary outcome measure of the GAIT study was a 20% decrease in knee pain. Analysis of the primary outcome measure showed that only the combination of glucosamine and chondroitin was efficacious for the reduction of pain, and only in those with moderate or severe OA[99]. Prior to the GAIT study, some investigations[100] had suggested efficacy of these component supplements (*Table 3.9*)[101–119].

Table 3.9 Influence of interleukin-1 (IL-1) on articular cartilage matrix components, inflammatory mediators, and degradative enzymes (Columns 3 and 4: note the + or – complementary effect from glucosamine and chondroitin sulfate). Numbers refer to supporting references

Mediator/matrix molecule	IL-1 effect on chondrocyte biosynthesis	Glucosamine effect	Chondroitin sulfate effect
	116–121	(+) inhibits, or (–) fails to inhibit effects induced by IL-1	(+) inhibits, or (–) fails to inhibit effects induced by IL-1
COX-2/PGE$_2$	Stimulates synthesis	+122, +123	+/–124–126
iNOS/NO	Stimulates synthesis	+122	+/–125
MMPs	Induces synthesis, activity, and secretion	+122, +127 +128	+126, +/–129
Aggrecanases/aggrecan	Increased synthesis and activity	+130, +131	
PGs GAGs	Decreased synthesis, increased degradation	+124	+124, +126, +132
Type II collagen	Inhibits synthesis	–124, –133	+124
Transcription factors (NFκB, AP 1)	Stimulates increased mRNA expression and activity	+123, +134	

Neil KM, Caron JP, Orth MW. The role of glucosamine and chondroitin sulfate in treatment for and prevention of osteoarthritis in animals. JAVMA 2005;**226**(7):1079–88[100].

Pharmacokinetic studies in dogs reveal that glucosamine hydrochloride is only 10-12% bioavailable from single or multiple doses[120]. At current recommended intake, it is extremely unlikely that relevant concentrations of glucosamine reach the joint[121], or that substantial amounts of glucosamine get into the circulation following oral ingestion[122]. Glucosamine is expected to be metabolized rapidly by the liver or incorporated into glycoproteins. Glucosamine is not ordinarily available in the circulation as a source of cartilage matrix substrate; cartilage uses glucose for that purpose. Charged molecules exceeding approximately 180 daltons are likely not to pass the GI mucosa and be absorbed unless assisted by a carrier-mediated transport system; therefore, it is unlikely that chondroitin sulfate would be absorbed intact via the GI tract. The gastric mucosa contains a number of GAG-degrading enzymes, such as exoglycosideases, sulfatases, and hyaluronidase-like enzymes, which should degrade chondroitin sulfate. Adebowale *et al.* reported the single oral dose bioavailability in dogs to be approximately 12% and 5% for glucosamine and chondroitin, respectively[120].

One rationale for using nutraceuticals is that provision of precursors of cartilage matrix in excess quantities may favour matrix synthesis and repair of articular cartilage. Glucosamine is an amino monosaccharide (2-amino-2-deoxy-α-D-glucose) that, once modified as N-acetylglucosamine, is proposed to act as a precursor of the disaccharide units of GAGs such as hyaluronan and keratan sulfate. Chondroitin sulfate is a GAG consisting of alternating disaccharide subunits of glucuronic acid and sulfated N-acetylgalactosamine. Substitution can occur at the C4 and C6 position of the sulfate residue attached to N-acetylgalactosamine to form chondroitin-4 sulfate and chondroitin-6 sulfate. Chondroitin sulfate is a normal constituent of cartilage; the ratio of C-4S to C-6S decreases with age. An alternative rationale for the use of glucosamine and chondroitin is that chondrocyte metabolism may be enhanced to produce aggrecan and collagen[123].

The literature contains some support for the use of glucosamine sulfate (GS) in humans. It has been observed that glucosamine hydrochloride does not induce symptomatic relief in knee OA to the same extent as GS[124]. Noteworthy is that GS is very hygroscopic and unstable, which is why varying amounts of potassium or sodium chloride are added during manufacturing. Dodge *et al.* reported that GS not only increased the expression of the aggrecan core protein but also down-regulated, in a dose-dependent manner, MMP-1 and -3 expression[125]. Some investigators have suggested that the metabolic contribution to OA cartilage from GS is associated with activation of protein kinase C, considered to be involved in the physiologic phosphorylation of the integrin subunit[126]. GS may restore fibrillated cartilage chondrocytes' adhesion to fibronectin, thus improving the repair process of OA cartilage by allowing proliferating cells to migrate to damaged areas. Support for both glucosamine and chondroitin sulfate mode of action is quite robust (**3.13**).

Glucosamine and chondroitin have both been long-standing popular nutraceuticals comprising the foundation of many supplements, and published data show a synergistic effect of their combined use (**3.14**): synergism being recognized as an improved effect of combined use, compared to either separate agent alone. Medicinal agent synergisms have become recognized for major advances in multimodal, mechanism-based disease treatments.

Avocado/soybean unsaponifiables

Avocado/soybean unsaponifiables (ASU) are a recent entry to the nutraceutical pool. It is suggested that this compound may promote OA cartilage repair by acting on chondrocytes and subchondral bone osteoblasts. ASU has been observed to prevent the inhibitory effect of subchondral osteoblasts on aggrecan synthesis while having no significant effect on MMP, tissue inhibiting metalloproteinase (TIMP-1), COX-2 or inducible nitric oxide synthetase (iNOS) expression[127]. In contrast, Henrotin *et al.* reported that ASU decreased MMP-3 production and stimulated TIMP-1 production, suggesting that ASU could have structure-modifying effects in OA by inhibiting cartilage degradation and promoting cartilage repair[128]. Additional studies support the role of ASU in abrogating various inflammatory mediators (**3.15**)[129-132]. The product Dasuquin® (Nutramax Laboratories Inc.) is an ASU-rich product.

Evidence indicating that joint diseases are associated with increased production of reactive oxygen species suggests that anti-oxidant agents

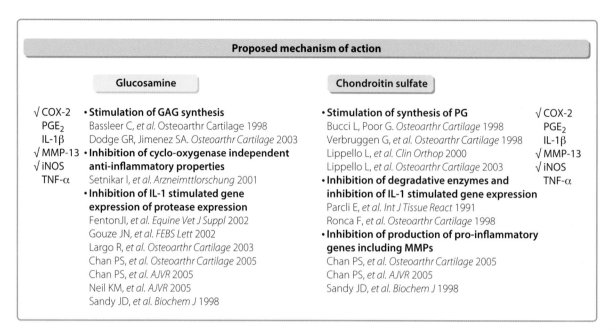

3.13 Support for both glucosamine and chondroitin sulfate mode of action is quite robust. Each agent has been reported to have both pro-anabolic and anti-catabolic or anti-inflammatory activities, with efficacy (√) in suppressing several major inflammatory mediators. GAG: glycosaminoglycan; PG: prostaglandin; IL: interleukin; MMP: matrix metalloproteinase; COX: cyclo-oxygenase; iNOS: inducible nitric oxide synthase; TNF: tumor necrosis factor.

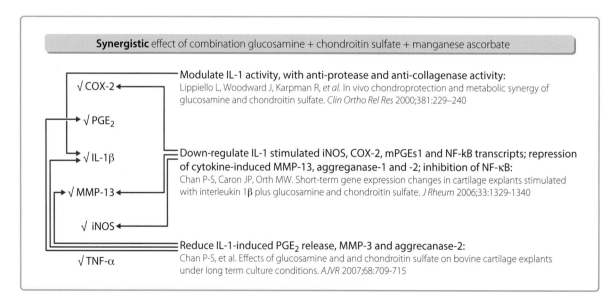

3.14 Synergism of combining glucosamine, chondroitin sulfate, and manganese ascorbate has shown improved *in vitro* effects in suppressing several major inflammatory mediators of osteoarthritis. GAG: glycosaminoglycan; PG: prostaglandin; IL: interleukin; MMP: matrix metalloproteinase; COX: cyclo-oxygenase; iNOS: inducible nitric oxide synthase; TNF: tumor necrosis factor NF-κB: nuclear factor kappa-light-chain-enhancer of activated B cells.

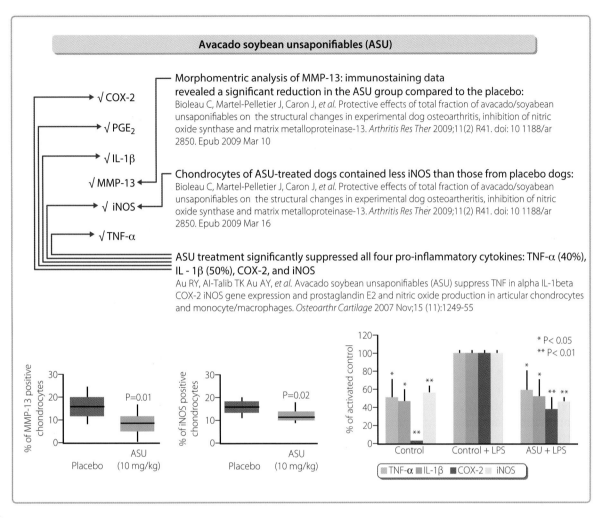

Avacado soybean unsaponifiables (ASU)

√ COX-2

√ PGE₂

√ IL-1β

√ MMP-13

√ iNOS

√ TNF-α

Morphomentric analysis of MMP-13: immunostaining data revealed a significant reduction in the ASU group compared to the placebo:
Bioleau C, Martel-Pelletier J, Caron J, *et al.* Protective effects of total fraction of avacado/soyabean unsaponifiables on the structural changes in experimental dog osteoarthritis, inhibition of nitric oxide synthase and matrix metalloproteinase-13. *Arthritis Res Ther* 2009;11(2) R41. doi: 10 1188/ar 2850. Epub 2009 Mar 10

Chondrocytes of ASU-treated dogs contained less iNOS than those from placebo dogs:
Bioleau C, Martel-Pelletier J, Caron J, *et al.* Protective effects of total fraction of avacado/soyabean unsaponifiables on the structural changes in experimental dog osteoartheritis, inhibition of nitric oxide synthase and matrix metalloproteinase-13. *Arthritis Res Ther* 2009;11(2) R41. doi: 10 1188/ar 2850. Epub 2009 Mar 16

ASU treatment significantly suppressed all four pro-inflammatory cytokines: TNF-α (40%), IL - 1β (50%), COX-2, and iNOS
Au RY, Al-Talib TK Au AY, *et al.* Avacado soybean unsaponifiables (ASU) suppress TNF in alpha IL-1beta COX-2 iNOS gene expression and prostaglandin E2 and nitric oxide production in articular chondrocytes and monocyte/macrophages. *Osteoarthr Cartilage* 2007 Nov;15 (11):1249-55

3.15 Avocado/soybean unsaponifiables (ASU) have shown *in vitro* effects in suppressing several major inflammatory mediators of osteoathritis. PG: prostaglandin; IL: interleukin; MMP: matrix metalloproteinase; COX: cyclo-oxygenase; iNOS: inducible nitric oxide synthase; TNF: tumor necrosis factor; LPS: lipopolysaccharide.

might have beneficial effects in the treatment of OA. Green tea contains the major anti-oxidant epigallo-catechin gallate (ECGC) and has become a popular nutraceutical beverage. ECGC has been shown to inhibit the onset and severity of collagen induced arthritis in mice[133,134.] Given the potential for synergism, in 2010 Heinecke and colleagues reported the combined effects of ASU and ECGC in equine chondrocytes[135].

The nuclear factor kappa-light-chain-enhancer of activated B cells (NF-κB) pathway plays a major role in inflammation, and considering the adage that 'inflammation is the mother of all disease', then NF-κB is to be recognized a major target for disease intervention. The increased expression of COX-2 and the concomitant increased production of PGE₂ resultant from disease cytokine-activation, makes COX-2 an important target for pharmacological intervention in treating OA. Heinecke, *et al.* (2010) have reported on the synergistic effect of ASU + EGCG in modulating COX-2, when administered prior to cytokine stimulation of equine chondrocytes *in vivo* (**3.16**)[135]. The synergistic relationship of ASU and EGCG is illustrated in **3.16** and **3.17**.

Alpha-lipoic acid (also known as ALA) is a synthetic version of lipoic acid, a naturally occurring compound produced in the body and synthesized by both plants and animals. This anti-oxidant is vital to cellular energy production, and helps to neutralize the damage caused by free radicals. Naturally occurring lipoic acid is always covalently bound and not readily available from dietary sources. In addition, the amount of lipoic acid present in dietary sources is very low. Studies suggest (**3.18**) that ALA is synergistic with ASU in suppressing PGE_2 production observed within inflammatory-stimulated cell cultures[136].

Boswellia is another nutraceutical of interest, based upon its historical medicinal use as an anti-inflammatory. The biblical incense frankincense is an extract from this tree's resin. Boswellia trees and shrubs are native to tropical regions of Africa and Asia. Extracts from both the resin and bark are used as tribal medicinals. Studies reveal that a proprietary *Boswellia serrata* extract works in synergism with ASU+glucosamine+chondroitin sulfate (**3.19**) to suppress the production of PGE_2 in IL-stimulated cell cultures[137].

Curcumin is yet another nutraceutical in common use (**3.20**). Turmeric (*Curcuma longa*) is a rhizomatous perennial plant of the ginger family, native to southwest India and Southeast Asia. One active ingredient of turmeric is curcumin, which is used as a spice condiment and has been used for thousands of years as a major part of Siddha medicine. Curcumin offers anti-inflammatory effects through inhibition of I kappa B kinase (IKK) of the NF-κB signalling pathway[138]. The anti-inflammatory role of curcumin is also mediated through down-regulation of COX-2 and iNOS through suppression of NF-κB activation[139-141].

Phycocyanin

Phycocyanin is composed of two protein subunits with covalently bonded phycobilins that are the light-capturing part of the blue pigment in blue–green algae. It is considered the active agent in PhyCox®, commercialized as PhyCox-JS®. However, there are some data suggesting that C-phycocyanin is a selective COX-2 inhibitor[142]. Phycocyanin has been shown to have anti-oxidant and anti-inflammatory properties *in vitro* and *in vivo* (rodents)[143,144]. Other ingredients in the product, which may contribute to product efficacy, include glucosamine, turmeric, EPA, and DHA. This product is not a drug, but positioned as an animal nutraceutical of natural

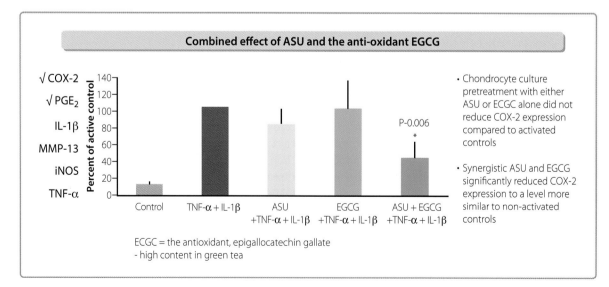

3.16 Avocado/soybean unsaponifiables (ASU) work synergistically with epigallocatechin gallate (EGCG) in suppressing the cyclo-oxygenase-2 (COX-2) response to inflammatory stimulation. PG: prostaglandin; IL: interleukin; MMP: matrix metalloproteinase; iNOS: inducible nitric oxide synthase; TNF: tumor necrosis factor.

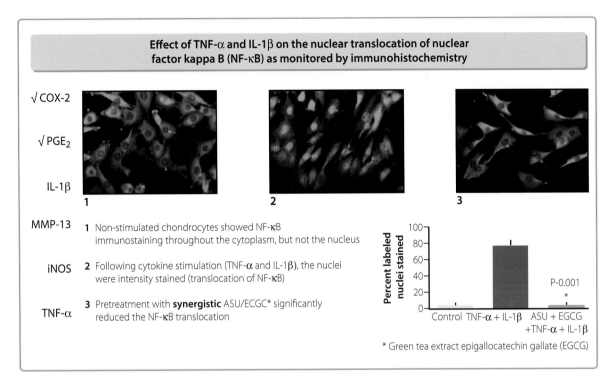

Effect of TNF-α and IL-1β on the nuclear translocation of nuclear factor kappa B (NF-κB) as monitored by immunohistochemistry

√ COX-2

√ PGE₂

IL-1β

MMP-13   1   Non-stimulated chondrocytes showed NF-κB immunostaining throughout the cytoplasm, but not the nucleus

iNOS   2   Following cytokine stimulation (TNF-α and IL-1β), the nuclei were intensity stained (translocation of NF-κB)

TNF-α   3   Pretreatment with **synergistic** ASU/ECGC* significantly reduced the NF-κB translocation

Control   TNF-α + IL-1β   ASU + EGCG +TNF-α + IL-1β

P-0.001

* Green tea extract epigallocatechin gallate (EGCG)

3.17 Cause and effect relationship between NF-κB nuclear translocation and up-regulation of COX-2 + PGE₂. With interleukin (IL)-1β/tumor necrosis factor (TNF)-α stimulation of equine chondrocytes, nuclear factor kappa-light-chain-enhancer of activated B cells (NF-κB) is translocated to the chrondrocyte nucleus as observed by immuostaining (2 vs. 1). Pretreatment of chondrocytes with the combination of avocado/soybean unsaponifiables (ASU) and epigallocatechin gallate (EGCG) prevents this translocation (3), resulting in the subsequent control of prostaglandin E2 up-regulation via its influence by cyclo-oxygenase (COX-2). PG: prostaglandin; IL: interleukin; MMP: matrix metalloproteinase; iNOS: inducible nitric oxide synthase.

3.18 Synergistically, alpha-lipoic acid (ALA) and avocado/soybean unsaponifiables (ASU) have been shown to suppress production of stimulated prostaglandin E₂ production by 20% greater than ASU alone. COX: cyclo-oxygenase; PG: prostaglandin; IL: interleukin; MMP: matrix metalloproteinase; iNOS: inducible nitric oxide synthase; TNF: tumor necrosis factor; LPS: lipopolysaccharide.

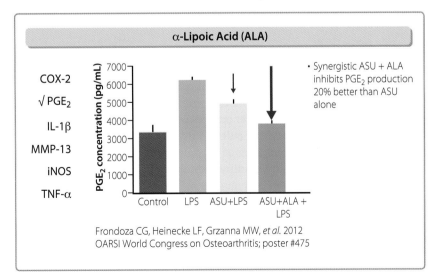

α-Lipoic Acid (ALA)

COX-2

√ PGE₂

IL-1β

MMP-13

iNOS

TNF-α

• Synergistic ASU + ALA inhibits PGE₂ production 20% better than ASU alone

Control   LPS   ASU+LPS   ASU+ALA + LPS

Frondoza CG, Heinecke LF, Grzanna MW, *et al.* 2012 OARSI World Congress on Osteoarthritis; poster #475

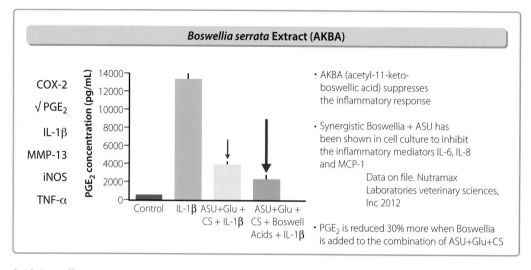

3.19 *Boswellia serrata* extract synergistically assists avocado/soybean unsaponifiables (ASU)+glucosamine+chondroitin sulfate (CS) to suppress prostaglandin E_2 (PGE_2) production from inflammatory-stimulated cell cultures. IL: interleukin; MMP: matrix metalloproteinase; iNOS: inducible nitric oxide synthase; TNF: tumor necrosis factor.

botanical origin. Its pharmacokinetics are unknown in the dog. The observational study performed by the manufacturer was based on owner observations of dogs on the ingredient C-phycocyanin and not the commercial product, and with no apparent control patients. Further, this product and other products classified as medical foods with purported anti-inflammatory activity have not been studied in use together with a NSAID. It is very possible that combining products with anti-inflammatory properties with NSAIDs may increase the incidence of ADEs.

Alternative to NSAID and opiate analgesics

The majority of emerging therapies for the treatment of moderate to severe pain are reformulations of existing pain medications combined with new delivery technologies that may offer only incremental improvements in efficacy and safety. Presently, the greatest need in the treatment of chronic pain is for agents that surmount the disadvantages of NSAIDs and opioid analgesics. Although great progress has been made in the efficacy of NSAIDs over the past couple of decades, safety is still an area of concern since patient potential for predisposition to ADEs (primarily gastrointestinal) is a 'craps shoot'. And, since painkiller addiction continues to spin out

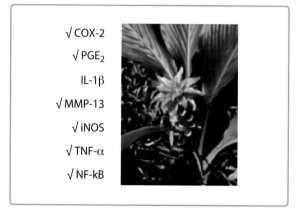

3.20 Curcumin appears to influence the nuclear factor kappa-light-chain-enhancer of activated B cells (NF-κB) pathway, thereby having anti-inflammatory effects through suppression of multiple degradative cytokines.

of control within our society, prescription opiate use is increasingly under scrutiny and regulatory constraint[145]. In the early 1900s, various viper venoms were under clinical assessment for the treatment of pain and epilepsy[146,147]. Several researchers established that cobra venom had cytotoxic properties which led to studies in patients with cancer, where its relief of pain was identified as the dominant pharmacodynamic activity[148].

The basis for cobra venom's activity is related to the principal neurotoxins comprising about 20–25% of the venom; with the primary receptor target being nicotinic acetylcholine receptors (nAchRs) associated with afferent neurons of nociception. nAchRs are sodium channels that are activated by acetylcholine and drugs, such as nicotine (agonists), that transpose chemical signals to action potentials for impulse conduction. They are blocked (antagonized through competitive inhibition) by neurotoxins such as those from cobras, because these neurotoxins have receptor affinities that are orders of magnitude greater than that of acetylcholine. Within the cholinergic system, nicotinic (and muscarinic) receptors contribute to modulating not only pain signals, but also inflammation and consequently inflammatory pain (giving rise to speculation that the sensation of pain may be augmented by acetylcholine-secreting cells that are external to the nervous system). At nonlethal doses, cobra venom is reported to ameliorate adjuvant-induced arthritis in rats[149], reducing not only pain but also tissue damage, confirming it as a potential disease-modifying antirheumatic drug for complementary and alternative medicine (CAM). Commonly, the onset of pharmacodynamic activity of peripherally administered cobra toxins is realized only after several hours in contrast to aspirin and morphine, but the activity is more prolonged[150–152].

Snake venoms are rich in nAChR neurotoxins[153], having shown analgesic effects in both human and animal pain models[154]. Such venoms contain α- and β-neurotoxins, acting through different mechanisms to block the transmission of acetylcholine and subsequent perception of pain in a number of animal species[151,153–155].

Alpha-neurotoxins act as nicotinic receptor antagonists by competitively binding to the nAChR at the postsynaptic membrane of both skeletal muscles and neurons, reversibly blocking nerve transmission[156]. Cobratoxin is a short-chain postsynaptic α-neurotoxin from the Chinese or Taiwan cobra, with high affinity for the muscle-based α1 subunit of the nAChR, while producing strong, centrally mediated analgesia. Cobratoxin is a long-chain postsynaptic α-neurotoxin from the Thailand cobra, with high affinity for the neuronal α7 subunit of the nAChR, located predominantly in the peripheral nervous system as well as in the brain. Additionally, α7nAChR regulates calcium ion channels, which in turn, modulate synaptic neurotransmitters. Owing to its anti-inflammatory and antinociceptive mechanisms, cobratoxin modulates the production of inflammatory cytokines and has analgesic properties in several animal species. The effects of cobratoxin are opiate-independent. Atropine affects cobratoxin activity, but naloxone does not[153].

A number of clinical trials assessing cobra venom analgesia have been reviewed[157], including one reported by Wang et al., wherein cobratoxin compared to morphine for postoperative pain management was found to act for twice as long as morphine, but with 150th the amount of drug on a per kg basis[158]. Cobra venom is a readily available, non-prescription, cost-effective resource analgesic. Cobra venom's historically impressive safety record and observed analgesic response rate warrant its consideration as an opiate alternative. The reported analgesic activity of cobra venom by oral administration has shown validity in animal models, where active agents gave equivalent analgesic effects to doses 300 times lower than aspirin and 30 times lower than morphine [proprietary data: Nutra Pharma, Coral Springs, FL]. The most common human side-effects are nausea and upset stomach.

Nutraceutical summary and recommendations

Many nutraceuticals are least-cost formulations and quality assurance is lacking to nonexistent[159,160]. As a matter of record, in 2005 the FDA rejected 12 model claims related to products reducing the risk of OA, joint degeneration, cartilage deterioration, and OA-related joint pain, tenderness, and swelling[161].

Controversy remains over mechanisms by which nutraceuticals may lead to modulation of disease signs and cartilage degradation in OA, and which product is preferred for treatment. Perhaps our scientific community lacks the expertise or financial support to identify how these products might work. Nevertheless, as a class of agents, nutraceuticals fall short in evidence-based efficacy, lack dose titration studies to validate appropriate doses of individual products, and have shown inconsistencies of product quality assurance. Good intentions of the few have been clouded by many! A sound recommendation for consumers is 'buyer beware'. One might argue that the most responsible advice for recommending a nutraceutical is as an adjunct to a 'science-based' medicinal, in that the nutraceutical may or may not help. Recommending that the pet owner administer a nutraceutical as the first line of treatment lacks convincing scientific underpinning, and product selection should be determined by the ACCLAIM criteria considering that all nutraceuticals are not created equal (see below)[162].

Nutramax Laboratories Inc., Edgewood, MD, USA consistently meets these criteria.

A-C-C-L-A-I-M criteria for selecting a nutraceutical

- A = A name you recognize?

Products manufactured by an established company that provides educational materials for veterinarians or other consumers are preferable to those manufactured by a new company.

- C = Clinical experience

Companies that support clinical research and have products used in clinical trials (e.g. safety, efficacy, or bioavailability studies) that are published in peer-reviewed journals to which veterinarians have access are more likely to have a quality product.

- C = Content

All ingredients should be clearly indicated on the product label.

- L = Label claims

Label claims that sound too good to be true probably are. Products with realistic label claims based on results of scientific studies, rather than testimonials, are more likely to be reputable. Products with illegal claims (i.e. claims to diagnose, treat, cure, or prevent a disease) should be avoided.

- A = Administration recommendations

Dosing instructions should be accurate and easy to follow; it should be easy to calculate the amount of active ingredient administered per dose per day.

- I = Identification of lot

A lot identification number or some other tracking system indicates that a premarket or postmarket surveillance system (or both) exists to ensure product quality. In addition, companies that have voluntarily instituted current good manufacturing practices and other quality-control or quality-assurance techniques (e.g. tamper-resistant packaging or identification of individual tablets or caplets) provide evidence of a long-term investment.

- M = Manufacturer information

Basic company information should be clearly stated on the label. Preferably, this should include a Web site or details for contacting customer support.

ADJUNCTS

OA is both a chronic disease and an acute disease, with intermittent flare-ups that may render a NSAID ineffective as a sole analgesic because of 'breakthrough pain'. Further, chronic pain is not just a prolonged version of acute pain. As pain signals are repeatedly generated, neural pathways undergo physiochemical changes that make them hypersensitive to the pain signals and resistant to antinociceptive input. In a very real sense, the signals can become embedded in the spinal cord, like a painful memory.

The main neurotransmitter used by nociceptors synapsing with the dorsal horn of the spinal cord is glutamate, a molecule that can bind to a number of different receptors. Discovering the role of the N-methyl-D-aspartatae (NMDA) receptor in chronic pain has given rise to the (empirical) implementation of NMDA antagonists, such as amantadine, which is occasionally administered together with voltage-gated ion channel modulator gabapentanoids as adjuncts in a multimodal OA protocol (also finding efficacy in other chronic pain diseases). When activated, the NMDA receptor site allows a massive intracellular influx of Ca^{++}, and subsequent neuronal release of neurogenic transmitters (**3.21**). The receptors and pathways involved in perception and transmission of noxious stimuli provide multiple sites for potential new analgesic drug development (**3.22, 3.23**).

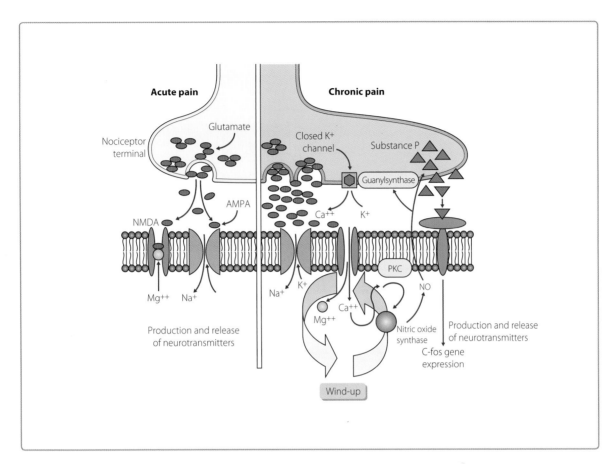

3.21 N-methyl-D-aspartate (NMDA) receptor activity plays a major role in differentiating acute from chronic pain. When activated the NMDA receptor site allows massive intracellular influx of Ca++, which initiates the state of 'wind-up'. AMPA: alpha-amino- 3-hydroxy-5-methyl-4- isoxazole propionic acid; PKC: protein kinase C.

3.22 N-methyl-D-aspartate (NMDA) facilitation amplifies the nociceptive signals to a state of hyperalgesia. Administration of an 'adjunct', such as an NMDA antagonist, blocks the NMDA-facilitated nociceptive signaling, suppressing the nociceptive signal back to a state of 'normalgesia'.

AMPA: alpha-amino- 3-hydroxy- 3-hydroxy-5-methyl-4- isoxazole propionic acid; CGRP: calcitonin gene related peptide; Glu: glutamate; NK-1: neurokinin-1; sP: substance P.

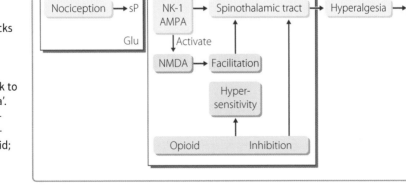

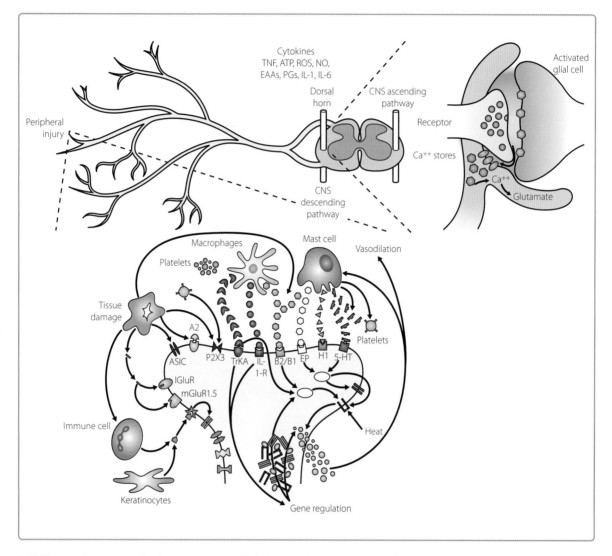

3.23 The moving target of pain management. Well characterized receptors in the periphery are activated by noxious stimuli, acute inflammation, and tissue injury, sending afferent information to the dorsal horn of the spinal cord where synaptic transmission to ascending pathways is subject to modulation by descending pathways, local neuronal circuits, and a variety of neurochemicals. Each of these receptors/modulators is a potential site for new analgesic drug development. A2: adenosine A2 receptor; ASIC: acid-sensing channels; ATP: adenosine triphosphate; B1/2: bradykinin receptors 1,2; EAAs: excitatory amino acids; EP: prostaglandin E receptor; H1: histamine H1 receptor; 5-HT: 5-hydroxytryptamine (serotonin); IGluR: ionotropic glutamate recceptor; IL: interleukin; IL-1R: interleukin 1 receptor; M2: muscarinic M2 receptor; mGluR: metabotropic glutamate receptor; NO: nitric oxide; P2X3: purinergic receptor X3; PAF: platelet-activating factor; ROS: reactive oxygen species; TrKA: tyrosine receptor kinase A.

Tramadol

The synthetic codeine analogue, tramadol is widely used (although not approved) in dogs. Approximately 40% of its activity is at the mu-receptor. Forty percent of tramadol activity is as a norepinephrine reuptake inhibitor and 20% is as a serotonin (5-HT) reuptake inhibitor (SRI) (**3.24**). Since tramadol has SRI features, its use can be associated with increased bleeding, especially when used in combination with an NSAID. Since the majority of tramadol activity is other than at the mu-receptor, it is a poor substitute for the 'pure' opioids; however, it can be used as an adjunct to an opioid or an NSAID[163]. In humans tramadol is able to reduce the amount of substance P in synovial fluid, as well as IL-6, which seems to correlate with the stage of OA[164]. The American College of Rheumatology and the American Medical Directors' Association support the addition of tramadol to an NSAID for the management of chronic pain in humans[165,166]. However, one meta-analysis on tramadol concluded that tramadol or tramadol/actaminophen decreases pain intensity, produces symptom relief, and improves function, but these benefits were small. Adverse events, although reversible and not life threatening, often caused participants to stop taking the medication and could limit its usefulness[167]. Despite its wide use, there is little to no safety or efficacy data on the use of tramadol in veterinary patients. Published data suggest caution with its cavalier use, pending further studies assessing its effects in cats and dogs[168,169].

Hyaluronic acid

Four potential mechanisms have been proposed for the beneficial clinical effects noted from hyaluronic acid (HA) therapy:

1. restoration of elastic and viscous properties of the synovial fluid[170].
2. biosynthetic–chondroprotective effect on cells (hyaluronans can induce endogenous synthesis of HA by synovial cells, stimulate chondrocyte proliferation, and inhibit cartilage degradation)[171,172].
3. anti-inflammatory effects[173,174].
4. analgesic effect[175,176].

HA acts as an aggregating factor between the collagen, PG aggregate, and cartilage structural network as a whole. Synovial fluid contains high concentrations of HA, derived from type B synoviocytes embedded within the intimal lining of the joint capsule. The viscoelastic properties of synovial fluid are determined by HA, and with the progression of OA, HA concentrations decrease with a resultant decrease in the viscoelastic properties of the synovial fluid. Intra-articular injection of HA, called viscosupplementation, has demonstrated significant improvement of symptoms in patients with OA[177]. By definition, injectable HA (e.g., Legend®) is not a nutraceutical. However, it can be considered a chondroprotective agent and there are several commercially available forms of HA, differing by treatment regimens, total dosing, and average molecular weights. Due to its molecular weight, HA is poorly absorbed by the gastrointestinal tract (5% in the dog) and consequently, it has been administered locally into the joint. In the rat, following oral administration, 0.5% reaches the knee joint[178].

In the joint, HA reaches synovial membranes by simple diffusion, and extracellular matrix of cartilage and subchondral bone through lymphatic flow[179]. Under physiological conditions, in the extracellular matrix HA is primarily found as high-molecular-weight HA (HMW-HA) (>500 kDa). HMW-HA promotes cell quiescence and tissue integrity by binding to receptors for pro-inflammatory

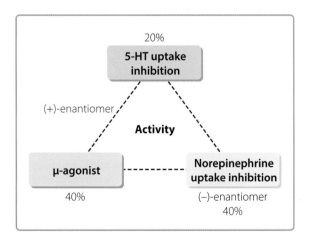

3.24 Tramadol is principally a tricyclic antidepressant with weak opioid-like features. 5-HT: 5-hydroxytryptamine.

signaling pathways[180]. Support for use of HA resides in the improvement of OA symptoms with few side-effects. It is unlikely that sustained beneficial effects of HA therapy result from temporary restoration of the synovial fluid lubrication and viscoelasticity[181]. Perhaps HA therapy has disease-modifying biological activity and an impact on OA progression.

ACUPUNCTURE

Acupuncture falls under the categorization of CAM as part of traditional Chinese medicine (TCM), and is used in humans in at least 78 countries worldwide[182]. From an historical perspective, little information about acupuncture was available in the USA until after President Richard Nixon's visit to China in 1972. However, in 1826 Benjamin Franklin's grandson, a Philadelphia physician, published that acupuncture was an effective treatment for pain associated with rheumatism and neuralgia among prisoners at the Pennsylvania state penitentiary[183]. It is a safe, low-cost modality which is easy to administer and has no side-effects if performed by a trained practitioner; it can be administered stand-alone or as a complement to other medical therapeutics. It is misleading to refer to a single universal form of traditional Chinese acupuncture, as there are more than 80 different acupuncture styles in China alone, in addition to many Japanese, Korean, Vietnamese, European, and American styles.

Theory of acupuncture
TCM places emphasis on function rather than structure. Accordingly, in such practice it is more important to understand the relationships between variables and the functional 'whole' of the patient than to identify the specifics of a single pathology. Basic to the practice of acupuncture is the yin–yang theory, where yin and yang are interdependent but possess similar characteristics (**3.25**)[184]. They can transform into each other, and can consume each other. In this regard, physiology and pathology are variations along a continuum of health and illness.

A common feature shared by all different types of acupuncture is using needles to initiate changes in the soft tissue. Needles and needle-induced changes are believed to activate the built-in survival mechanisms that normalize homeostasis and promote self-healing. Herein, acupuncture can be defined as a physiologic therapy coordinated by the brain, which responds to the stimulation of manual or electrical needling of peripheral sensory nerves, where acupuncture does not treat any particular pathologic system, but normalizes physiologic homeostasis and promotes self-healing[185]. Acupuncture can be effective for both peripheral soft tissue pain and internal disorders, but in the case of peripheral soft tissue pain the result appears more predictable because of the local needle reaction.

Hypotheses of acupuncture mechanisms
The leading hypotheses include the effects of local stimulation, neuronal gating, the release of endogenous opiates, and the placebo effect. It is further proposed that the CNS is essential for the processing of these effects via its modulation of the autonomic nervous system, the neuroimmune system, and hormonal regulation. Clinical observation suggests that acupuncture needling achieves at least four therapeutic goals: 1) release of physical and emotional stress; 2) activation and control of immune and anti-inflammatory mechanisms; 3) acceleration of tissue healing; and 4) pain relief secondary to endorphin and serotonin release.

Keeping in mind that acupuncture therapy is considered to activate built-in survival mechanisms, i.e. self-healing potential, it is effective for those symptoms that can be completely or partially healed by the body. Additionally, each individual has a different self-healing capacity influenced by genetic makeup, medical history, lifestyle, and age, all of which may be dynamically changing.

Ancient Chinese thought holds that Qi is a fundamental and vital substance of the universe, with

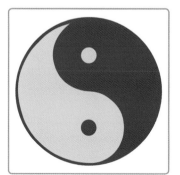

3.25 Symbolic representation of the yin–yang theory, where yin and yang are interdependent and possess similar characteristics.

all phenomena being produced by its changes. It is considered a vital substance of the body, flowing along organized pathways known as acupuncture channels, or meridians, helping to maintain normal activities. TCM suggests that a balanced flow of Qi throughout the system is required for good health, and acupuncture stimulation can correct imbalances. As of the mid-1990s, stimulation of acupuncture points is believed to cause biochemical changes that can affect the body's natural healing. The primary mechanisms involved in these changes include enhanced conduction of bioelectromagnetic signals, activation of opioid systems, and activation of autonomic and central nervous systems causing the release of various neurotransmitters and neurohormones[186]. Approximately 30 years ago it was discovered that acupuncture analgesia could be reversed by naloxone, a pure antagonist to all known opioids[187]. Acupuncture can change concentrations of serotonin and biogenic amines, including opioid peptides, met-enkephalin, leu-enkephalin, α-endorphin, and dynorphin.

Acupuncture can also be explained, in part, by Melzack and Wall's Gate Theory. When large, myelinated A-δ and A-β fibers are stimulated by acupuncture, impulses from small unmyelinated C-fibers, transmitting ascending nociceptive information, are blocked by a gate of inhibitory interneurons. The strongest evidence for acupuncture efficacy in human cancer has been in the areas of nausea, vomiting, and pain control[188,189].

Kapatkan et al. reported that electrostimulated acupuncture did not have any significant effects on severity of lameness, as determined by measurement of ground reaction forces, or severity of pain, as determined by visual analog scale pain scores, in dogs with chronic elbow joint OA secondary to elbow joint dysplasia[190].

RADIOSYNOVIORTHESIS (RADIO-SYNOVI-ORTHESIS): A NEW THERAPEUTIC AND DIAGNOSTIC TOOL FOR CANINE JOINT INFLAMMATION

John M. Donecker, VMD, MS and
Nigel R. Stevenson, PhD

Synovial inflammation is strongly implicated in the pathogenesis of OA and other arthropathies. Synovitis is a common feature of symptomatic but pre-radiographic OA. This indicates that chronic, early-stage joint inflammation occurs well before significant radiographic changes and drives progression toward cartilage loss, osteophyte formation, bone remodeling, and joint space narrowing[191,192,193]. The pathology of early-onset synovitis and its role in OA have been well characterized. Whereas normal synovium is two or three cell layers thick and devoid of inflammatory cells, synovitis results in a number of profound changes in synovial tissue and the joint micro-environment. These include marked hyperplasia and permeability of the synovial lining, significant over-expression of proinflammatory mediators and cytokines, infiltration of inflammatory cells, production of degradative enzymes, synovial neo-vascularization, and increased serum C-reactive protein, a biomarker of inflammation[194,195,196]. The inflammatory response sensitizes peripheral neurons in synovial tissue, resulting in a pain response[197].

OA should not be thought of as a single entity, but as a sequence of events beginning with joint injury followed by synovitis and progressing to OA as the clinical endpoint[192]. The demonstration that significant synovitis precedes structural changes in the progression of OA indicates that early intervention targeting pre-radiographic joint inflammation can delay or prevent chronic arthritic changes[193]. Surgical and non-surgical synovectomy (synoviorthesis) have been used for relieving synovitis in human, canine, and equine patients. Herein, the focus is on radiosynoviorthesis (RSO) using a homogenous colloid radiolabeled with tin-117m, a novel radionuclide that offers significant advantages over conventional radionuclides.

Definitions

beta particle: A high-energy electron emitted from the nucleus of a radioactive atom; beta particles typically have a wide tissue penetration range of 50–5,000 μm that diminishes over distance, making uniform dosing difficult and possibly necessitating shielding during transport and handling.

colloid: A mixture of insoluble micro particles (particles between 0.1 to 100.0 μm in size) that remain distributed in solution without precipitating or settling to the bottom; non toxic colloids are used for binding radionuclides to prevent them from escaping the intra-articular space into systemic distribution.

conversion electrons: Low-energy electrons released from an atomic shell as a result of radioactive decay, resulting when gamma radiation emitted by the nucleus is transferred to an electron; conversion electrons are monoenergetic in contrast to beta particles.

homogenous tin-117m colloid (HTC): A novel preparation of the radionuclide tin-117m suspended in a colloid; HTC is well suited for intra-articular administration to treat synovial inflammation caused by traumatic injury, OA, and other athritides.

radiocolloid: A radionuclide-labeled colloid suitable for intra-articular injection.

radionuclide: An unstable isotope of an atom that emits radiation released from the atomic nucleus. Some radionuclides exist naturally but those with research and therapeutic applications are usually produced artificially. A radioisotope.

radiosynovectomy (RSV): Refers to removal of the synovium and its replacement with fibrotic tissue, for example when joints are injected with beta-emitting radionuclides with a wide tissue-penetration range. Historically, RSV has been used interchangeably though less accurately as a synonym for RSO.

radiosynoviorthesis (RSO): Injection into the synovial space of a radioisotope to treat joint inflammation and mitigate chondromalacia when systemic or other traditional therapies have failed to produce a satisfactory response. The goal of RSO is a reduction of synovitis characterized by pain and synovial hypertrophy.

synovectomy: Destruction or surgical removal of the membrane (synovium) that lines an articular joint. Open surgical, chemical, radiation, and arthroscopic synovectomies are all options for removing potentially damaging synovium from articular joints.

synoviorthesis: A medical therapy using intra-articular injection of a compound that diminishes the degree of synovial hypertrophy, thereby mitigating pain and the development of inflammation and arthritis. Can be performed by chemical synoviorthesis or radiosynoviorthesis, with the latter being preferred when a suitable radionuclide is available.

tin-117m (Sn-117m): An artificially produced radionuclide of tin with medical applications for localized treatment and imaging. Tin-117m has a half-life of 14 days. Two principal forms of the energy that it emits are 1) conversion electrons that have a short penetration range in tissue (~300 μm), and 2) imageable gamma radiation, which enables monitoring of local distribution in tissue. Tin-117m is metastable, indicated by the 'm' suffix, meaning that it is a radioisotope with an energetic nucleus and a relatively long half-life and therefore distinct from highly unstable radionuclides with shorter half-lives.

Radiosynoviorthesis for intra-articular therapy

RSO has been successfully used in human medicine for more than 60 years in many countries, particularly in Europe where it was first described and where its use conforms to guidelines published by the European Association of Nuclear Medicine[198–201]. RSO has been an accepted outpatient therapy for treatment of early stage chronic synovitis in rheumatoid arthritis, psoriatic arthritis, and OA patients for decades[200,202]. RSO has important advantages versus surgical resection, the oldest ablative method. For example, as a minimally invasive procedure, RSO lowers bleeding risk in cases of hemophilic synovitis, where it is routinely used[203,204]. As a localized treatment, RSO avoids problems associated with systemic therapies such as toxicity resulting from chronic use of NSAIDs or immunosuppressive drugs. RSO also avoids tissue degradation that can occur from overuse of intra-articular corticosteroids. In human medicine, RSO has a favorable cost–benefit ratio, particularly when compared to surgery, a low rate of side-effects and application to virtually all articular joints, especially small, peripheral joints such as the phalangeal joints[200]. Current standards in human clinical practice generally take a conservative approach by recommending initial treatment with front-line therapies including systemic NSAIDs, glucocorticoids, and local joint therapies such as corticosteroid and HA injections prior to RSO[199]. However, in patients that either respond poorly or have adverse side effects following these traditional therapies, RSO is a useful option that is now being considered in veterinary medicine.

Radiosynoviorthesis in clinical practice

The term RSO was introduced in Europe in the 1960s by Florian Delbarre to describe therapeutically active irradiation of the synovial lining[198]. Rheumatologists administered a colloid embedded with a radionuclide (i.e. a radiocolloid) of yttrium-90 (90Y) into the articular space. Using this process, the colloidal particles are phagocytized by macrophages in the synovial lining, after which they emit therapeutically active irradiation of the synovial tissue until the radionuclide decays to its stable state. The number of inflammatory cells causing synovitis is reduced and inflamed tissue is replaced with a fibrotic synovial membrane, with a corresponding alleviation of pain and improvement in function[199,200]. An early study of RSV using beta-emitting samarium-153 in horses had mixed results, producing effective synovectomy but with transient lameness and swelling and exposure of some non-targeted, periarticular tissue[205].

A key aspect of RSO is the choice of a radionuclide. Three radionuclides are widely used in clinical practice to treat synovitis: 90Y, rhenium-186 (186Rh),

and erbium-169 (169Er), all of which are artificially produced in a nuclear reactor[199-201]. In the case of RSO treatment, the radionuclide emits radiation that penetrates the outermost layer of the synovial membrane where it produces energy of sufficient duration and intensity to achieve apoptosis and ablation of the inflamed cells. For this to occur, the radionuclide must have an adequate half-life (t½), a selective tissue penetration range approximating the synovial thickness, and sufficient energy for therapeutic effect.

As 90Y, 186Rh, and 169Er decay, they emit radiation in the form of beta particles with a relatively wide tissue penetration range[198-201]. While these radionuclides are therapeutically useful and have been evaluated in large clinical trials[199], their physical properties are not necessarily ideal for RSO. For example, 90Y emits beta radiation that has a relatively wide range of soft tissue penetration, which risks irradiation of adjacent non-synovial tissue. 186Re and 90Y have short half-lives (2.7 and 3.7 days, respectively), which create storage and logistical limitations and may not consistently deliver sufficient irradiation at the synovial target site[204].

Tin-117m: A novel radionuclide

Tin-117m is a unique radionuclide without the disadvantages of high-energy beta-emitting radionuclides (*Table 3.10* compares physical properties of tin-117m with other therapeutic radionuclides). As such, tin-117m is particularly well suited for RSO, including in dogs and horses. Instead of high-energy beta particles with a wide tissue penetration range

Table **3.10** Comparison of radionuclides commonly used for radiosynoviorthesis[206].

Radionuclide	Half-life (days)	Maximum energy (keV)	Maximum tissue penetration (mm)	Therapeutic emission	Diagnostic emission (keV)
Yttrium-90	2.7	2,280	11.0	beta	None
Rhenium-186	3.7	1,070	4.4	beta	gamma (201)
Erbium-169	9.4	350	1.1	beta	None
Tin-117m	13.6	158	0.3	conversion electrons	gamma (209)

keV = kilo-electron volt.

(50–5,000 μm), tin–117m emits abundant conversion electrons (**3.26**, see Definitions), a low-energy particle with a short penetration range of approximately 300 μm in tissue[198–201]. Tin-117m has a t½ of nearly 14 days, providing an ideal duration of effect spanning several half-lives to achieve therapeutic results and to enable short-term stability during storage and handling. To illustrate, there is >99% dose retention in the joint of a dog (**3.27**) 3 days following intra-articular injection with HTC[206]. No other radionuclide with the properties of tin-117m exists[207].

In addition to conversion electrons, tin-117m emits gamma radiation, a zero-mass quantum of light and electromagnetic radiation that results from nuclear decay of a radionuclide. Gamma radiation is non-therapeutic but readily detectable in tissue by imaging methods such as scintigraphy. By emitting gamma radiation at 159 kilo-electron volts (keV), tin-117m can be used diagnostically to detect the distribution and duration of its presence in tissue of treated patients. This application is similar to that for technetium-99m (99mTc), a widely used systemic radionuclide with gamma emissions of 140 keV that is used in diagnostic procedures, including evaluation of bone structure and function.

Due to its unique therapeutic and diagnostic (theranostic) properties as a conversion electron- and gamma-emitter with an optimal t½, tin-117m has attracted interest as a radiopharmaceutical and also now as a medical device in the colloid form. Favorable results were reported in phase I and II clinical trials where tin-117m was used to treat metastatic bone pain in human patients[208–210]. Investigators noted the value of the gamma emission component of tin-117m, which provides an objective basis for diagnostic monitoring, disease staging, dosage estimates, and assessing response to therapy[210,211].

A homogenous colloid of tin-117m

R-NAV, LLC has developed a patented preparation of tin-117m specifically for RSO and other potential

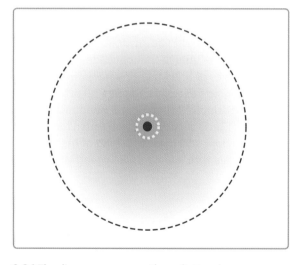

3.26 The diagram compares the radiation dose range of conversion electrons emitted by Tin-117m (300 μm, green zone) with beta-radiation emitted by radionuclides such as yttrium-90 and erbium-169 (50–5,000 μm, blue zone). The ultra-narrow, discrete radiation range of tin-117m enables more precise dosimetry and avoidance of adverse effects on adjacent tissues such as can occur with beta-emitting radionuclides.

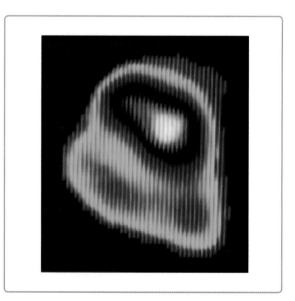

3.27 Scintigraphy of an homogenous tin-117m colloid (HTC)-injected canine elbow shows high dose-retention of the homogenous colloid with minimal uptake in the draining lymph node three days after administration. Retention at this time point was measured at >99% in synovial tissue, indicating a continuous therapeutic effect consistent with the 14-day half-life of tin-117m. (Image courtesy of Jimmy Lattimer, DVM.)

applications in veterinary and human medicine. Tin-117m is manufactured using methods that produce yields sufficient to be scaled up for manufacturing therapeutic dosages in commercial quantities[207]. The tin-117m radionuclide is combined with a homogenous colloid[207]. The radionuclide particles are small enough to be phagocytized by synovial macrophages but large enough to avoid leakage outside the joint prior to phagocytosis. *In situ* retention of the HTC in laboratory animals has been measured out to five t½ (i.e., 70 days), a duration sufficient for therapeutic efficacy. The HTC has demonstrated safety and efficacy following RSO of experimental OA in rats and dogs and safety in normal canine elbow joints (**3.28**).

Clinically important features of tin-117m

Several features of tin-117m make it well suited for RSO and an improvement over other therapeutic radionuclides:

- Localized administration: Intra-articular dosing is suitable for outpatient use.
- Non-beta emitter: Avoids high-energy irradiation of non-synovial tissue, extra-articular diffusion, or systemic distribution.
- Emits low-energy conversion electrons: Minimizes potential for synovial scarring and eliminates collateral tissue damage.
- Gamma radiation emitter: Gamma energy of 159 keV is suitable for diagnostic imaging and is similar to the commonly used diagnostic radionuclide Tc-99m (140 keV).
- Half-life of 14 days: Enables sufficient tissue retention for therapeutic efficacy and a shelf life of 5 weeks.
- Practical handling characteristics: Ease of handling, hospital containment, and shipping using standard radiological safety and packaging practices.

Radiosynoviorthesis in veterinary medicine

Radiotherapy has had various applications in companion animal medicine. For example, the beta-emitter iodine-131 (^{131}I) has been used systemically to treat feline hyperthyroidism since the 1990s and is considered the treatment of choice for that condition[211]. Palliative and curative radiation therapy is now commonly used at veterinary

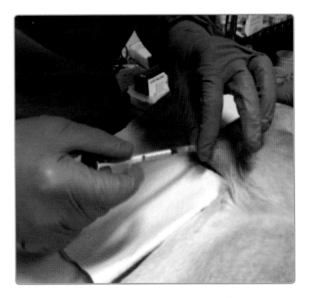

3.28 Experimental intra-articular injection of the radionuclide tin-117m into the caudo-lateral aspect of a canine elbow, positioned at 45-degree flexion, between the lateral condyle of the humerus and the triceps tendon. Following injection the joint is put through a range of motion to disperse the radiocolloid throughout the synovial surface. (Photo courtesy of Cynthia Doerr, MD.)

oncology referral centers[212], and radionuclides are also used for bone scanning in animals. Not surprisingly, successful RSO in human patients has created interest in using this method in companion animals and horses as a treatment for synovitis. Experimental RSO in horses has been attempted at university centers both in Europe and in the USA[205,213,214]. Investigators in those studies used the beta-emitting radionuclides holmium-166 (166Ho) or samarium-153 (153Sm). However, high-energy emissions from either radionuclide resulted in some transient, periarticular soft-tissue injury and minor extra-articular joint leakage[205,213,214]. In a small Australian study, 90Y was administered concurrently with methylprednisolone acetate to four horses with severe chronic synovitis and hemarthrosis[215]. Median return to normal joint use was 7 months, with two of the horses developing recurrent hemarthrosis.

In experimental studies with thulium-170 and 90Y, healthy dogs were used as models for comparing results of canine and human RSO[216-218]. Results indicated that RSO in dogs is feasible and generally well tolerated. However, the studies found that excessive dosages of beta-emitting radionuclides can reduce glycosaminoglycan synthesis in articular cartilage and result in extra-articular leakage of radiocolloid particles as late as 9 months after intra-articular administration. Such outcomes reflect the importance in clinical applications of using well characterized radionuclides that emit radiation within well-defined parameters. Successful RSO in relatively small canine joints was noteworthy given the commonplace occurrence of canine elbow dysplasia and associated OA, a small-joint pathology that would be difficult to treat surgically[219].

A safe and effective RSO radionuclide

Based on widespread clinical and experimental experience with beta-emitting radionuclides, a safe and effective radiocolloid suitable for RSO has the following characteristics[199,210]:

- A limited, discrete emission penetration depth that corresponds to the thickness of the synovium (i.e. avoids irradiation too shallow for clinical effect or that extends beyond the synovial layer to affect non-target tissue).
- An intermediate radionuclide t½ that is long enough to provide a reasonable shelf life and to produce a therapeutic effect but short enough to avoid excessive exposure.
- A homogenous colloid that binds the radionuclide so that it cannot escape beyond the joint.
- Suitable colloid particle size for synovial phagocytosis and *in situ* retention.
- Gamma emission for purposes of diagnostic imaging.
- Large production yields that allow scaling up for cost-effective manufacturing.
- A clinical profile that demonstrates a high degree of efficacy and safety.

Because non-beta emitting HTC satisfies all of these criteria, it is considered to be uniquely suited for RSO treatment[207]. Further evaluation in canine, feline, and equine models is expected to affirm its suitability for synovitis treatment combined with diagnostic confirmation of therapeutic response.

DRUG CLASSES FOR MULTIMODAL USE

A popular combination for multimodal use consists of drugs from the opioid and NSAID classes (*Table 3.11*). This combination is commonly used postoperatively and for addressing the World Health Organization's cancer pain ladder recommendation for mild-to-moderate and moderate-to-severe pain. There are several opioid/NSAID combination drugs commercially available for human use (*Table 3.12*), although they are not commonly used in veterinary medicine (*Table 3.13*) due to differences in dosages, tablet size requirements, and safety issues .

Table 3.11 Comparison of opioid and NSAID pharmacology

	Opioids	NSAIDs
Mechanism	Predominantly central	Predominantly peripheral
Availability	Controlled substances	Noncontrolled/some available OTC
Therapeutic ceiling	No	Yes
Tolerance	Yes	Unlikely
Addiction	Possible	Not possible
GI side-effects: nausea and vomiting	More frequent	Less frequent
constipation	Frequent	No
gastric ulceration	No	Possible
GI bleeding	No	Possible
Respiratory side-effects	Depression	Infrequent
Effects on pupil	Yes	No
Cognitive impairment	Yes	No

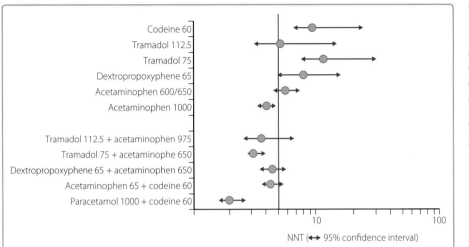

3.29 Number needed to treat (NNT) (humans) comparing single-dose combinations and their components. NNT is an estimate of the number of patients that would need to be given a treatment for one patient to achieve a desired outcome (e.g. 50% pain relief over 4–6 hr). Generally NNT 2–5 are indicative of effective analgesic treatments[176].

Number needed to treat (NNT) is a common scheme for comparing human analgesic drug efficacy (**3.29**)[220]. Edwards et al. showed that the analgesic efficacy of the nonopioid analgesics is improved (in humans) by combination with weak opioids[221].

NONMEDICINAL MANAGEMENT

Nonmedical management consists of three principal aspects (**3.30**): diet, weight control, and physical rehabilitation.

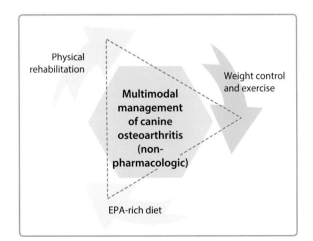

3.30 Nonmedicinal management of osteoarthritis consists of weight control and exercise, eicosapentaenoic acid (EPA)-rich diet, and physical rehabilitation (as required).

Table 3.12 Some NSAID*–opioid commercial drug combinations available for human use

Combination	Trade name	Strength (mg)
Aspirin + caffeine + dihydrocodeine	Synalgos	356.4 + 30 + 16
Aspirin + carisoprodol + codeine	Soma compound w/codeine	325 + 200 + 16
Aspirin + codeine	Empirin w/codeine #3 Empirin w/codeine #4	325 + 30 325 + 60
Aspirin + hydrocodone	LortabASA	500 + 5
Aspirin + oxycodone	Persodan-Demi Percodan	325 + 2.25 325 + 4.5
Ibuprofen + oxycodone	Combunox	400 + 5
Ketoprofen + hydrocodone	Vicoprofen	200 + 7.5
Aspirin + caffeine + propexyphene HCl	Darvon compound -65	389 + 32.4 + 65

* Acetaminophen is not included in this table because acetaminophen is not technically a NSAID: it has analgesic properties, but not anti-inflammatory properties.

Table 3.13 Drugs commonly used together in multimodal protocols

Opioid	Dose	Species	Route	Duration	Comments
Morphine	0.5–1.0 mg/kg	Canine	IM, SC, IV	3–4 hr	Caution with IV administration: histamine release; give slowly
	0.05–0.1 mg/kg	Feline	IM, SQ	3–4 hr	
	0.2 mg/kg: loading, IM	Canine: 0.1–0.5 mg/kg/hr Feline: 0.05–0.1 mg/kg/hr	IM then CRI (IV)		
	0.1 mg/kg preservative-free	Canine/Feline	Epidural	12–24 hr	
	1–5 mg in 5–10 ml saline	Canine	Intra-articular		
Meperidine	3–5 mg/kg	Canine/Feline	IM, SC	1–2 hr	Do NOT give IV (histamine release)
Methadone	0.1–0.5 mg/kg	Canine/Feline	IM, SC, IV	2–4 hr	NMDA antagonist activity
Oxymorphone	0.05–0.1 mg/kg 0.03–0.05 mg/kg	Canine Feline	IM, IV, SQ IM, SQ	3–4 hr 3–4 hr	Minimal histamine release
Hydromorphone	0.1–0.2 mg/kg	Canine/Feline	IM, IV, SQ	2–4 hr	Minimal histamine release; hyperthermia may be seen in cats
Fentanyl	5 µg/kg + 3–6 µg/kg/hr 2–3 µg/kg + 2–3 µg/kg/hr	Canine Feline	IV IV	Infusion Infusion	
Fentanyl patch	25 µg/hr	Canine: 3–10 kg		1–3 days	24 hr to reach peak concentrations
	50 µg/hr 75 µg/hr 100 µg/hr 25–50 µg/hr	Canine: 10–20 kg Canine: 20–30 kg Canine: >30 kg Feline		1–3 days 1–3 days 1–3 days ≤6 days	6 hr to reach peak concentrations

Opioid (cont.)	Dose	Species	Route	Duration	Comments
Butorphanol (10 mg/ml)	0.1–0.2 mg/kg 0.2–0.4 mg/kg IV; then 0.1–0.2 mg/kg/hr	Canine/Feline Canine/Feline	IM, IV, SQ CRI	Canine: 1 hr Feline: 2–4 hr	Low oral bioavailability
Pentazocine	1–3 mg/kg	Canine/Feline	IM, IV, SQ	2–4 hr	
Nalbuphine	0.03–0.1 mg/kg	Canine/Feline	IM, IV, SQ	2–4 hr	
Buprenorphine	10–30 µg/kg	Canine/Feline	IM, IV, SQ	4–10 hr	15–30 min onset. Excellent buccal mucosa absorption in cats
Tramadol	2–10 mg/kg (suggested) 5 mg/kg (suggested)	Canine Feline	PO PO	6–8 hr	Nonscheduled. Mu agonist activity. Serotonin and norepinephrine reuptake inhibitor. NMDA antagonist at lower doses, GABA receptor inhibitor at high concentrations
Codeine	1–2 mg/kg	Canine	PO	4–6 hr	
Alpha-2 agonist					
Medetomidine / Dexmedetomidine	2–15 µg/kg 5–20 µg/kg 1 µg/kg IV; then 1–2 µg/kg/hr 1–5 µg/kg 2–5 µg/kg	Canine Feline Canine/Feline Canine/Feline Canine/Feline	IM, IV IM, IV CRI Epidural IA	0.5–1.5 hr 0.5–1.5 hr	Sedation, bradycardia, vomiting
Xylazine	0.1–0.5 µg/kg	Canine/Feline	IM, IV	0.5–1.0 hr	
Yohimbine (antagonist)	0.1 mg/kg IV; 0.3–0.5 mg/kg IM	Canine/Feline			
Atipamezol (antagonist)	0.05–0.2 mg/kg IV	Canine/Feline			2–4 times the medetomidine dose volume

(Table 3.13 continued on next page)

Table 3.13 *(Continued)*

NMDA antagonist	Dose	Species	Route	Duration	Comments
Ketamine	0.5 mg/kg IV; then 0.1–0.5 mg/kg/hr	Canine/Feline	CRI		
Amantadine	3–5 mg/kg	Canine/Feline	PO	24 hr	Neuropathic pain
Dextro-methorphan	0.5–2 mg/kg	Canine	PO, SQ, IV		D-isomer of codeine; weak NMDA antagonist NOT RECOMMENDED due to side-effects[157]
Methadone	0.1–0.5 mg/kg	Canine/Feline	IM, SC	2–4 hr	Opioid derivative
Tricyclic antidepressant					
Amitriptyline	1.0 mg/kg	Canine	PO	12–24 hr	Enhanced noradrenergic activity
	0.5–1.0 mg/kg	Feline	PO	12–24 hr	
Ca++ channel modulator					
Gabapentin	5–10 mg/kg	Canine/Feline	PO	12–24 hr	Voltage dependent Ca++ channel inhibitor
Adjunct					
Acepromazine	0.025–0.05 mg/kg	Canine	IM, SQ, IV	8–12 hr	3 mg maximum total dose; used to potentiate or prolong analgesic drug effect
	0.05–0.2 mg/kg	Feline	IM, SQ	8–12 hr	
Diazepam	0.1–0.2 mg/kg	Canine/Feline	IV	2–4 hr	Used to potentiate or prolong analgesic drug effect
	0.25–1.0 mg/kg	Canine/Feline	PO	12–24 hr	

Local anesthetics	Dose	Species	Route	Duration	Comments
Lidocaine (1–2%)	≤6.0 mg/kg	Canine	Perineural	1–2 hr	Onset: 10–15 min. Maximum dose: 12 mg/kg (canine); 6 mg/kg (feline)
	≤3.0 mg/kg 2–4 mg/kg IV, then 25–80 µg/kg/min	Feline Canine	Perineural IV: CRI	1–2 hr	
	0.25–0.75 mg/kg slow IV, then 10–40 µg/kg/min	Feline	IV: CRI		NOTE: efficacy and safety are not yet convincing
Bupivacaine (0.25–0.5%)	≤2.0 mg/kg	Canine	Perineural	2–6 hr	Onset: 20–30 min. Maximum dose: 2 mg/kg (canine or feline)
	≤1.0 mg/kg	Feline	Perineural	2–6 hr	
Mepivacaine (1–2%)	≤6.0 mg/kg ≤3.0 mg/kg	Canine Feline	Perineural Perineural	2–2.5 hr 2–2.5 hr	

Kukanich B, Papich MG. Plasma profile and pharmacokinetics of dextromethorphan after intravenous and oral administration in healthy dogs. *J Vet Pharmacol Ther* 2004;**27**:337–41.

DIET

Diet is arguably one of the most important environmental factors influencing health and disease. Although genes are critical for determining predilections, nutrition modifies the extent to which different genes are expressed and thereby modulates whether individuals fully express the promise established by their genetic background. New genomic technologies, the so called '-omics tools', are now elucidating the basis of the associations between diet and health. These technologies monitor the activity of multiple genes simultaneously at the level of ribonucleic acid (RNA) by transcriptomics, the level of the proteins by proteomics, and, ultimately, the level of metabolites by metabolomics. The science of nutrigenomics employs all of these tools to clarify how nutrients influence health and disease by altering the expression of an individual's genetic makeup (**3.31**)[222]. The application of nutrigenomics to specific veterinary conditions is opening new avenues of disease prevention and therapy[223]. The role of n-3 fatty acids in canine OA is one example of application of nutrigenomic principles to clinically important conditions in veterinary medicine.

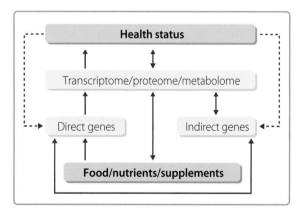

3.31 Nutrition can affect gene expression both directly and indirectly. Changes in gene expression are reflected in the transcriptome, proteome, and metabolome.

Weight control

Impellizeri *et al.* showed that in overweight dogs with hind limb lameness secondary to hip OA, weight reduction alone may result in a substantial improvement in clinical lameness[14]. Further, from the Labrador Retriever life-long Nestlé Purina study, Kealy and others showed that the prevalence and severity of OA in several joints were less in dogs with long-term reduced food intake compared with control dogs fed *ad libitum*, and that food intake is an environmental factor that may have a profound effect on the development of OA in dogs (**3.32**)[15,16]. Dogs on a restricted diet showed a significant reduction in progression of OA hip scores and lived longer (**3.33**). Over the life-span of investigated dogs, the mean age at which 50% of the dogs required long-term treatment for clinical signs attributable to OA was significantly earlier (10.3 years, p<0.01) in the overweight dogs as compared to the dogs with normal body condition scores (13.3 years)[15].

Adipocytes

Traditionally the mechanical stress of excess weight has been thought to be a primary perpetrator of the pathophysiology and progression of OA. However, recent studies have documented metabolic activity in adipose tissue that may be of equal or greater importance. Adipocytes secrete several hormones including leptin and adiponectin, and produce a diverse range of proteins termed adipokines. Among the currently recognized adipokines is a growing list of mediators of inflammation: tumor necrosis factor (TNF)-α, IL-6, IL-8, and IL-10 (**3.34**). These adipokines have been documented in both human and canine adipocytes[224,225]. Production of these proteins is increased in obesity, suggesting that obesity is a state of chronic low-grade inflammation. The presence of low-grade inflammation may contribute to the pathophysiology of a number of diseases commonly associated with obesity, including OA. This might explain why relatively small reductions in

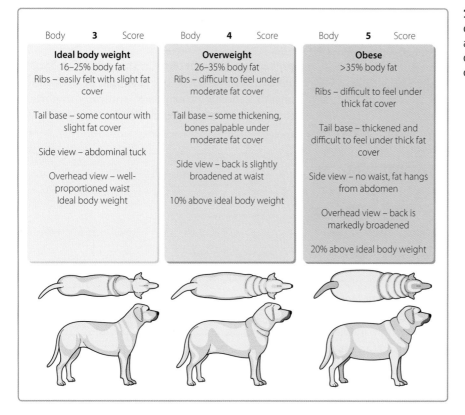

Body **3** Score	Body **4** Score	Body **5** Score
Ideal body weight	**Overweight**	**Obese**
16–25% body fat	26–35% body fat	>35% body fat
Ribs – easily felt with slight fat cover	Ribs – difficult to feel under moderate fat cover	Ribs – difficult to feel under thick fat cover
Tail base – some contour with slight fat cover	Tail base – some thickening, bones palpable under moderate fat cover	Tail base – thickened and difficult to feel under thick fat cover
Side view – abdominal tuck	Side view – back is slightly broadened at waist	Side view – no waist, fat hangs from abdomen
Overhead view – well-proportioned waist	10% above ideal body weight	Overhead view – back is markedly broadened
Ideal body weight		20% above ideal body weight

3.32 Dogs with body condition scores >3/5 are at increased risk for developing clinical signs of osteoarthritis.

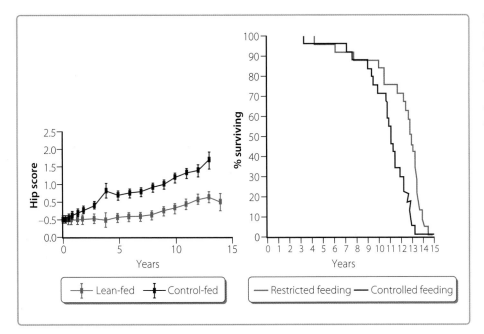

3.33 Dogs on a diet of restricted caloric intake not only demonstrate a significant reduction in progression of osteoarthritis hip scores but also live longer.

body weight can result in significant improvement in clinical signs[14]. The overproduction of inflammatory mediators in obese individuals is associated with changes in the genome. These changes may enhance the phenotypic expression of OA compared to genetically similar dogs that remain lean their entire lives.

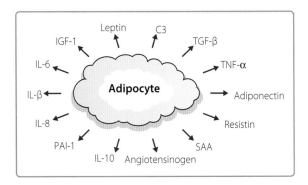

3.34 Hormones, cytokines, and other growth substances secreted from adipose tissue. This list continues to grow as new substances are identified. C3: complement protein 3; IGF-1: insulin-like growth factor-1; IL: interleukin; PAI-1: plasminogen activator inhibitor-1; SAA: serum amyloid A; TNF-α: tumor necrosis factor-α; TGF-β: transforming growth factor-β.

The structure–function relationship of articular cartilage

Aggrecan is the major proteoglycan (by mass) of articular cartilage, consisting of the proteoglycan monomer that aggregates with hyaluronan. Many aggrecan monomers attach to a hyaluronic acid chain to form an aggrecan aggregate. Aggrecan aggregates, type II collagen fibrils, water, and chondrocytes comprise the cartilage matrix (**2.2**) wherein structure reflects function. When structure is altered, so too is function.

A disruption in the normal relationship of collagen and proteoglycans in the articular cartilage matrix is one of the first events in the development of OA. Compared with normal cartilage, OA-affected chondrocytes behave like an activated macrophage, with up-regulation of IL-1, IL-6, and IL-8 gene expression. Also up-regulated in arthritic chondrocytes are PGE$_2$, TNF-α, nitric oxide, and MMP-2, -3, -9, and -13.

These enzymes, MMPs, and aggrecanases destroy collagen and proteoglycans faster than new ones can be produced, transitioning the cartilage from an anabolic state to a catabolic state. An imbalance of TIMPs and MMPs contributes to the pathologic breakdown of cartilage.

The influence of substrate on eicosanoid production

AA and EPA act as precursors for the synthesis of these inflammatory cytokines, including PGs and leukotrienes, which are also known as eicosanoids. The amounts and types of eicosanoids synthesized are determined by the availability of the fatty acid precursor and by the activities of the enzyme systems that synthesize them. In most conditions the principal precursor for these compounds is AA, although EPA competes with AA for the same enzyme systems. The eicosanoids produced from AA are proinflammatory. In contrast, eicosanoids derived from EPA promote minimal to no inflammatory activity. Ingestion of oils containing n-3 fatty acids results in a decrease in membrane AA levels. This produces an accompanying decrease in the capacity to synthesize eicosanoids from AA. Studies have documented that levels of inflammatory eicosanoids produced from AA are depressed when dogs consume foods with relatively high levels of n-3 fatty acids[226].

Resolution of inflammation

Reducing the production of proinflammatory mediators is only one mechanism by which n-3 fatty acids promote reduced inflammation and the return to homeostasis. In people, failure to resolve inflammation has emerged as a central component of many diseases in modern western civilization (e.g. arthritis, periodontal disease, cardiovascular disease, cancer, and Alzheimer's disease)[227]. Recent work has demonstrated that resolution of inflammation is an active endogenous process aimed at protecting the individual from an excessive inflammatory response. The first endogenous local counter-regulatory mediators recognized were the lipoxins, which are derived from AA (**3.35**)[228]. More recently, two new families of lipid mediators derived from omega-3 fatty acids, resolvins and protectins, have been identified. These bioactive mediators have potent anti-inflammatory, neuroprotective, and proresolving properties[226]. Further elucidation of the molecular actions of these previously unappreciated families of lipid-derived mediators may shed light on the clinically recognized beneficial effects of omega-3 fatty acids. Although the molecular mechanisms for controlling the resolution of inflammation through resolvins and protectins have not been fully elucidated, it is conceivable that omega-3 fatty acids modulate this process at the level of the genome or proteome (**3.36**). The end result is that when the omega-3 fatty acid EPA replaces AA in cell membranes, the inflammatory cascade is decreased. Further, dog chondrocytes selectively store EPA (and no other omega-3 fatty acid) in the chondrocyte membrane, which turns off signal mRNA that prompts production of degradative aggrecanase (**3.37**).

Clinical studies indicate that nutritional management using a therapeutic food supplemented with n-3 fatty acids helped improve the clinical signs of

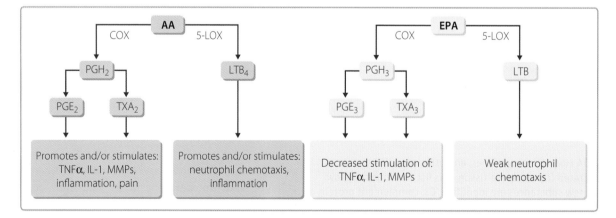

3.35 Types of eicosanoids synthesized are determined by the availability of the fatty acid precursor. LT: leukotriene; AA: arachidonic acid; PG: prostaglandin; TX: thromboxane; TNF: tumor necrosis factor; IL: interleukin; MMP: matrix metalloproteinase.

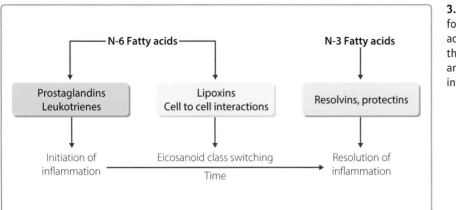

3.36 Proposed mechanism for n-6 and n-3 fatty acid-derived mediators in the initiation, transition, and resolution of acute inflammation.

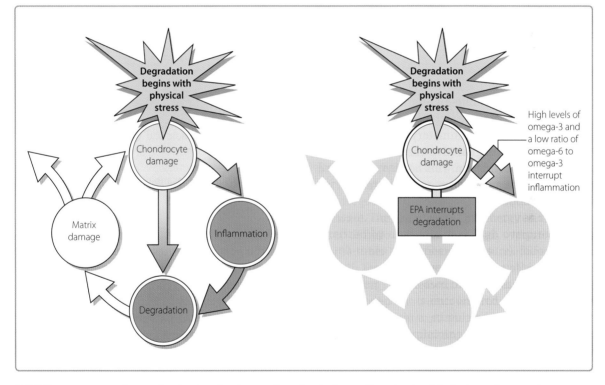

3.37 The common pathways that lead to the destruction of articular cartilage begin with the loss of proteoglycans (aggrecans). Damage to chondrocytes causes up-regulation of catabolic enzymes, particularly aggrecanases. Aggrecanase enzymes destroy proteoglycans faster than new ones can be synthesized. This imbalance leads to deterioration of the extracellular matrix, and cartilage's normal physiologic properties, and ultimately to structural and functional failure of the joint. In canine cartilage, eicosapentaenoic acid (EPA) has been shown to inhibit the up-regulation of aggrecanase enzymes by blocking the signal at the level of the messenger RNA, thereby interrupting the self-perpetuating cycle of degradation. By replacing arachidonic acid in cell membranes, EPA also modulates the inflammatory response.

OA in dogs as noted by pet owners, clinical ortho-pedic examination, and gait analysis of ground reaction forces. Clinical trial results from feeding EPA-rich diets have demonstrated increased serum EPA concentrations, improved clinical performance as assessed by both the veterinarian and pet owner, improved weight bearing as measured by force plate gait analysis, and have shown effective NSAID dose reduction[229].

Based on these studies, a food designed to aid in the management of OA in dogs should provide levels of total omega-3 fatty acids of 3.5–4.5% (dry matter) and specifically 0.41–1.1% (dry matter) EPA. The n-6 to n-3 fatty acid ratio should be less than 1:1. Dogs consuming the therapeutic food should receive an average of 55–100 mg EPA/kgBW/day. These results demonstrate that therapeutic foods developed through the application of nutrigenomic principles can result in clinically significant improvements in patients suffering from OA.

In summary, EPA diets have two principal modes of action: 1) by providing an alternative substrate for COX and lipoxygenase metabolism, the resultant prostanoids are less inflammatory; and 2) EPA diets help suppress the degradative enzymes associated with cartilage destruction. This helps maintain the integrity of hyaline cartilage, and subsequently its function (**3.38, 3.39**).

Understanding the relationship between genes, nutrients, and health is the central tenet of nutrigenomics. As this emerging field matures it is reasonable to envision an era where dietary intervention, based on knowledge of nutritional requirements, nutritional status, and genotype can be used to prevent or cure chronic disease. It has been suggested that, in the future, nutrigenomics may well hold the key to ensuring optimal health and longevity for both humans and animals regard-less of their genetic predispositions.

Physical rehabilitation

Physical rehabilitation is fast becoming an import-ant component of a multimodal approach to treating OA. Physical rehabilitation is a term that defines a broad spectrum of methods from the most advanced techniques used in complex orthopedic surgery recoveries to the simple techniques that can be taught to pet owners for use at home with their

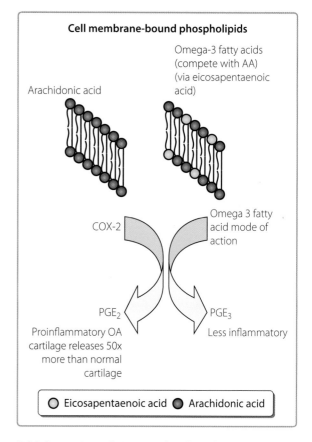

3.38 Comparison of eicosanoid end-products as influenced by substrate. AA: arachidonic acid; COX: cyclo-oxygenase; PG: prostaglandin; OA: osteoarthritis.

pets. The goal is to restore, maintain, and promote optimal function, optimal fitness, wellness, and quality of life as they relate to movement disorders and health.

The chronic OA patient is often reluctant to exercise. This reluctance may be due to the patient's unwillingness or inability. Unwillingness is frequently due to pain, which can be managed pharmacologically. However, the inability is often a consequence of decreased muscle mass and decreased joint range of motion, both the sequelae of OA. Physical rehabilitation focuses on the patient's inability to exercise, providing a resultant 'freedom of movement', and serves as a palliation of the disease progression. Frequently, physical reha-bilitation together with weight control can be as effective as, or more effective, than pharmacologic intervention.

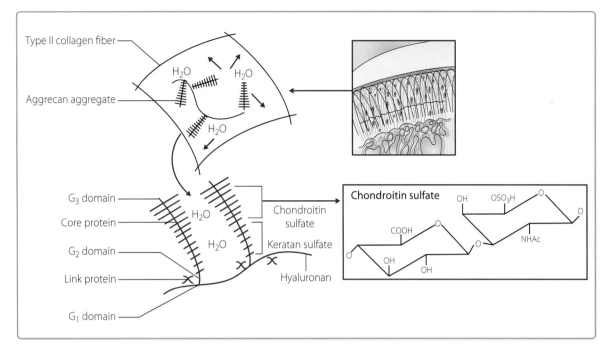

3.39 The aggrecan aggregate is the functional unit of articular cartilage, and articular cartilage is a tissue wherein structure is directly associated with function. Dietary eicosapentaenoic acid (EPA) suppresses the up-regulation of the aggrecanase enzyme, thereby sparing the integrity of the aggrecan aggregate, and sparing the function of articular cartilage.

SURGICAL INTERVENTION

The focus of this textbook is on the 'conservative' management of degenerative joint disease. However, it must be recognized that surgical intervention is necessary for some patients. Surgery most often involves extraction of inciting causes (e.g. ununited anconeal process [UAP], fragmented coronoid process [FCP], joint mouse osteophytes, osteochondritis dissecans [OCD] lesions) and/or attempts to stabilize an affected joint. Clear indications for surgery include, but are not limited to:

- Cruciate ligament deficient stifle and/or meniscal tears.
- Symptomatic medial or lateral patellar luxation.
- FCP and UAP.
- Hip dysplasia that is nonresponsive to 'conservative management'.
- End stage: tarsal or carpal disease, stifle disease, hip disease, and elbow disease.

- Chronic shoulder luxation.
- OCD lesions.

SUMMARY

The term multimodal has come to denote the co-utilization of different delivery modes, a variety of different drug class agents, and various techniques, the objective of which is to provide the patient with a minimal effective dose of each agent and therefore render optimal pain relief with minimal risk for adverse response (**3.40**). Specifically regarding NSAIDs, the cornerstone of treatment for OA, a multimodal approach encourages responsible use. 'Best medicine' dictates the clinician's responsibility to achieve a minimal effective dose for each patient. Registered labeling regarding dosage makes this more easily achieved with some NSAIDS than with others.

Following adoption of the multimodal scheme, the question at hand is sequencing the different modalities. Herein, there appear to be two different suggestions (**3.40**). Some suggest starting the patient on nonpharmacologic modalities, such as nutraceuticals, weight loss, and diet modifications (dotted line). Thereafter, the pharmacologic agents are integrated. However, this approach is challenged by two well-founded arguments. First, it is recognized that most of the nonpharmacologic modalities take 3–4 weeks before a clinical response is observed, and pet owners want to see a response sooner than that. Second, it is in the patients' best interest to provide analgesia as soon as possible. Anything less could be argued as inhumane, not providing immediate relief to the patient which it needs and deserves. Accordingly, the solid line path would appear the most ethical.

REFERENCES

1 Aragon CL, Hofmeister EH, Budsberg SC. Systematic review of clinical trials of treatments for osteoarthritis in dogs. *JAVMA* 2007;**230**:514–21.

2 Sanderson RO, Beata C, Flipo R-M, *et al.* Systematic review of the management of canine osteoarthritis. *Vet Record* 2009;**164**(14):418–24.

3 Millis DL. Nonsteroidal anti-inflammatory drugs, disease-modifying drugs, and osteoarthritis. *Supplement to Veterinary Medicine*, 2006, pp.9–19

4 Millis DL, Weigel JP, Moyers T, *et al.* Effect of deracoxib, a new COX-2 inhibitor, on the prevention of lameness induced by chemical synovitis in dogs. *Vet Ther* 2002;**24**:7–18.

5 Vasseur PB, Johnson AL, Budsberg SC, *et al.* Randomized, controlled trial of the efficacy of carprofen, a nonsteroidal anti-inflammatory drug, in the treatment of osteoarthritis in dogs. *JAVMA* 1995;**206**:807–11.

6 Peterson KD, Keef TJ. Effects of meloxicam on severity of lameness and other clinical signs of osteoarthritis in dogs. *JAVMA* 2004;**225**:1056–60.

7 Lust G, Williams AJ, Burton-Wurster N, *et al.* Effects of intramuscular administration of glycosaminoglycan polysulfates on signs of incipient hip dysplasia in growing pups. *Am J Vet Res* 1992;**53**:1836–43.

8 De Haan JJ, Goring RL, Beale BS. Evaluation of polysulfated glycosaminoglycan for the treatment of hip dysplasia in dogs. *Vet Surg* 1994;**23**:177–81.

9 Sevalla K, Todhunter RJ, Vernier-Singer M, *et al.* Effect of polysulfated glycosaminoglycan on DNA content and proteoglycan metabolism in normal and osteoarthritic canine articular cartilage explants. *Vet Surg* 2000;**29**:407–14.

10 Millis DL, Korvick D, Dean D, *et al.* 45th Meeting ORS 1999, p. 792.

11 Kukanich B, Papich MG. Pharmacokinetics of tramadol and the metabolite O-desmethyltramadol in dogs. *J Vet Pharmacol Ther* 2004;**27**:239–46.

12 Emkey R, Rosenthal N, Wu SC, *et al.* Efficacy and safety of tramadol/acetaminophen tablets (Ultracet) as add-on therapy for osteoarthritis pain in subjects receiving a COX-2 nonsteroidal anti-inflammatory drug: a multicenter, randomized, double-blind, placebo-controlled trial. *J Rheumatol* 2004;**31**:150–6.

13 Bennett GJ. Update on the neurophysiology of pain transmission and modulation: focus on the NMDA-receptor. *J Pain Symptom Manage* 2000 www.hosppract.com 2000 (discontinued).

14 Impellizeri JA, Tetrick MA, Muir P. Effect of weight reduction on clinical signs of lameness in dogs with hip osteoarthritis. *JAVMA* 2000;**216**(7):1089–91.

15 Kealy RD, Lawler DF, Ballam JM, *et al.* Five-year longitudinal study on limited food consumption and development of osteoarthritis in coxofemoral joints of dogs. *JAVMA* 1997;**210**(2):222–5.

16 Kealy RD, Lawler DF, Ballam JM, *et al.* Evaluation of the effect of limited food consumption on radiographic evidence of osteoarthritis in dogs. *JAVMA* 2000;**217**(11):1678–80.

17 Kealy RD, Lawler DF, Ballam JM, *et al.* Effects of diet restriction on life span and age-related changes in dogs. *JAVMA* 2002;**220**:1315–20.

18 Kealy RD, Olsson SE, Monti KL, *et al.* Effects of limited food consumption on the incidence of hip dysplasia in growing dogs. *JAVMA* 1992;**201**:857–63.

19 Burkholder WJ, Taylor L, Hulse DA. Weight loss to optimal body condition increases ground reaction forces in dogs with osteoarthritis. Purina Research Report 2000.

20 Johnston SA, Budsberg SC, Marcellin-Little D, *et al.* Canine osteoarthritis: overview, therapies,

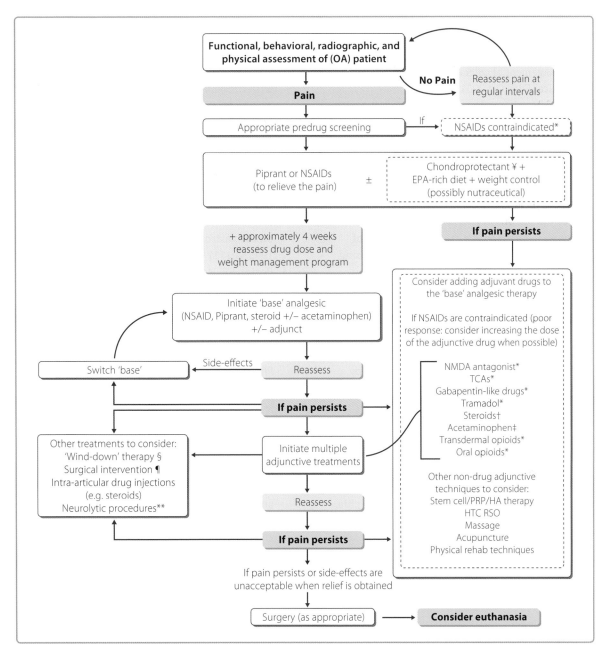

3.40 Algorithm for implementing a multimodal approach for osteoarthritis (OA) patients.* These drugs may be used in combination without a nonsteroidal anti-inflammatory drug (NSAID), acetaminophen, or a steroid base, but are likely to be less effective. †Steroids should not be used in combination with a NSAID. ‡Acetaminophen has been used in combination with NSAIDs, but it probably increases the risk of gastrointestinal ulceration. §'Wind-down' therapy refers to an unproven technique of using combinations of intravenous analgesics over a 48–72–hour period in OA cases that are refractory to oral treatment in an attempt to 'wind-down' the central nervous system changes and allow oral treatment to be more effective. ¶Surgical intervention refers to total hip or other joint replacement and arthrodesis. **'Neurolytic' is used to refer to surgical denervation and also neuroablative procedures. ¥= Adequan®Canine (polysulfated glycosaminoglycan). (Modified from Lascelles 2009 Merial Pain Management Symposium 2009 NAVC Conference and 2009 Western Veterinary Conference.). NSAID: nonsteroidal anti-inflammatory drug; PRP: platelet-rich plasma; HA: hyaluronic acid; RSO: radiosynoviorthesis. EPA: eicosapentaenoic acid; TCA: tricyclic antidepressant; NMDA: N-methyl-D-aspartate.

& nutrition. NAVC Clinician's Brief, April 2005; Supplement.

21   Waldron M. The role of fatty acids in the management of osteoarthritis. Nestlé Purina Clinical Edge Oct 2004, pp. 14–16.

22   IAMS. Nutrition plays a key role in joint health. Study finds that proactive nutrition can minimize use of NSAIDs. IAMS Partners for Health, July 2003; V1, No.3.

23   Laflamme DP. Fatty acids in health and disease. Nestlé Purina Research Report **10**(2):2006.

24   Bauer JE. Responses of dogs to dietary omega-3 fatty acids. *JAVMA* 2007;**231**:1657–61.

25   Innes JF, Caterson B, Little CB, *et al.* Effect of omega-3 fatty acids on canine cartilage: using an in vitro model to investigate therapeutic mechanisms. 13th ESVOT Congress 2006, Munich.

26   Levine D, Millis DL, Marcellin-Little D, *et al. Vet Clin North Am (SAP)*, 2005;**35**. WB Saunders, Philadelphia.

27   Millis DL, Levine D, Brumlow M, *et al.* A preliminary study of early physical therapy following surgery for cranial cruciate ligament rupture in dogs. VOS 1997, Big Sky MT.

28   Marcellin-Little D. Multimodal management of osteoarthritis in dogs. Symposium: a multimodal approach to treating osteoarthritis. Western Veterinary Conference 2007 Las Vegas.

29   Millis D, Levine D, Taylor RA. *Canine Rehabilitation & Physical Therapy*. WB Saunders, Philadelphia, 2004.

30   Lascelles BDX, Blikslager AT, Fox SM, *et al.* Gastrointestinal tract perforations in dogs treated with a selective cyclooxygenase-2 inhibitor: 29 cases (2002–2003). *JAVMA* 2002;**227**(7):1112–17.

31   3-Year Deramaxx Update. Novartis Animal Health USA, Inc. 2007: DER 060058A 35618.

32   Warner TD, Mitchell JA. Cyclooxygenase-3 (COX-3): filling in the gaps toward a COX continuum? *Proc Natl Acad Sci USA* 2002;**99**:13371–3.

33   Wallace JL, Keenan CM, Gale D, *et al.* Exacerbation of experimental colitis by nonsteroidal anti-inflammatory drugs is not related to elevated leukotriene B4 synthesis. *Gastroenterology* 1992;**102**(1):18–27.

34   Martel-Pelletier J, Mineau F, Fahmi H, *et al.* Regulation of the expression of 5-lipoxygenase-activating protein/5-lipoxygenase and the synthesis of leukotrienes B4 in osteoarthritic chondrocytes. *Arthritis Rheumatol* 2004;**50**:3925–33.

35   Pharmacovigilance summary: clinical experience with Deramaxx (deracoxib) since its US Launch. *Advisor for the Practicing Veterinarian* 2004 (DER 030103A).

36   Lascelles BDX, McFarland JM. Guidelines for safe and effective use of nonsteroidal anti-inflammatory drugs in dogs. *Technical Bulletin*, Pfizer Animal Health. November 2004.

37   Dow SW, Rosychuk RA, McChesney AE, *et al.* Effects of flunixin and flunixin plus prednisone on the gastrointestinal tract of dogs. *Am J Vet Res* 1990;**51**:1131–8.

38   Boston SE, Moens NM, Kruth SA, *et al.* Endoscopic evaluation of the gastroduodenal mucosa to determine the safety of short-term concurrent administration of meloxicam and dexamethasone in healthy dogs. *Am J Vet Res* 2003;**64**:1369–75.

39   De Leon-Casasola OA (ed). *Cancer Pain. Pharmacologic, interventional, and palliative approaches*. WB Saunders, Philadelphia, 2006, p. 284.

40   Hampshire VA, Doddy FM, Post LO, *et al.* Adverse drug event reports at the United States Food and Drug Administration Center for Veterinary Medicine. *JAVMA* 2004;**225**:533–6.

41   Cheng HF, Harris RC. Renal effects of nonsteroidal anti-inflammatory drugs and selective cyclooxygenase-2 inhibitors. *Curr Pharm Des* 2005;**11**:1795–1804.

42   Cohen HJ, Marsh DJ, Kayser B. Autoregulation in vasa recta of the rat kidney. *Am J Physiol* 1983;**245**:F32–F40.

43   Pages JP. Nephropathies dues aux anti-inflammatores non steroidiens (AINS) chez le chat: 21 observations (1993–2001). *Prat Med Chir Anim Comp* 2005;**40**:177–81.

44   Papich MG. An update on nonsteroidal anti-inflammatory drugs (NSAIDs) in small animals. In: Mathews KA (ed.) *Veterinary Clinics of North America. Small Animal Practice. Update on Management of Pain.* 2008;**38**(6):

45   Harvey JW, Kaneko JJ. Oxidation of human and animal haemoglobins with ascorbate, acetylphenylhydrazine, nitrite, and hydrogen peroxide. *Br J Haematol* 1976;**32**:193–203.

46 Dowers KL, Uhrig SR, Mama KR, *et al.* Effect of short-term sequential administration of nonsteroidal anti-inflammatory drugs on the stomach and proximal portion of the duodenum in healthy dogs. *Am J Vet Res* 2006;**67**(10):1794–1801.

47 Dahl G, Dahlinger L, Ekenved G, *et al.* The effect of buffering of acetylsalicylic acid on dissolution, absorption, gastric pH and faecal blood loss. *Int J Pharm* 1982;**10**:143–51.

48 Phillips BM. Aspirin-induced gastrointestinal microbleeding in dogs. *Toxicol Appl Pharmacol* 1973;**24**:182–9.

49 Singh G, Triadafilopoulos G. Epidemiology of NSAID-induced GI complications. *J Rheumatol* 1999;**26**(Suppl):18–24.

50 Morton DJ, Knottenbelt DC. Pharmacokinetics of aspirin and its application in canine veterinary medicine. *J SA Vet Assoc* 1989;**60**(4):191–4.

51 Price AH, Fletcher M. Mechanisms of NSAID-induced gastroenteropathy. *Drugs* 1990;**40**(Suppl 5):1–11.

52 Christoni A, Lapressa F. Richerche farmacologiche sull aspirina. *Arch Farmarol* 1909;**8**:63. Cited by Ghross M, Greenburg LA. In: *The Salicylates*. Hillhouse Press, New Haven, 1948.

53 Boulay JP, Lipowitz AJ, Klausner JS. The effect of cimetidine on aspirin-induced gastric hemorrhage in dogs. *Am J Vet Res* 1986;**47**:1744–6.

54 Hurley JW, Crandall LA. The effects of salicylates upon the stomachs of dogs. *Gastroenterology* 1964;**46**:36–43.

55 Taylor LA, Crawford LM. Aspirin-induced gastrointestinal lesions in dogs. *JAVMA* 1968;**152**(6):617–19.

56 Lipowitz AJ, Boulay JP, Klausner JS. Serum salicylate concentrations and endosopic evaluation of the gastric mucosa in dogs after oral administration of aspirin-containing products. *Am J Vet Res* 1986;**47**(7):1586–9.

57 Nap RC, Breen DJ, Lam TJGM, *et al.* Gastric retention of enteric-coated aspirin tablets in beagle dogs. *J Vet Pharmacol Ther* 1990;**13**:148–53.

58 Radi ZA, Khan NK. Review: Effects of cyclooxygenase inhibition on bone, tendon, and ligament healing. *Inflamm Res* 2005;**54**:358–66.

59 Trepanier LA. Potential interactions between nonsteroidal anti-inflammatory drugs and other drugs. *J Vet Emerg Crit Care* 2005;**15**(4):248–53.

60 Goodman L, Trepanier L. Potential drug interactions with dietary supplements. *Compendium (SAP)* October 2005, pp. 780–9.

61 US Pet Ownership and Demographics Sourcebook. *AVMA*, 2007. (www.avma.org/ reference/ marketstats/ownership.asp).

62 Lascelles BDX, Court MH, Hardie EM, *et al.* Nonsteroidal anti-inflammatory drugs in cats: a review. *Vet Anaesth Anal* 2007;**34**:228–50.

63 Hardie EM, Roe SC, Martin FR. Radiographic evidence of degenerative joint disease in geriatric cats: 100 cases (1994–1997). *JAVMA* 2002;**220**:628–32.

64 Franks JN, Boothe HW, Taylor L, *et al.* Evaluation of transdermal fentanyl patches for analgesia in cats undergoing onychectomy. *JAVMA* 2000;**217**:1013–20.

65 Lascelles BDX, Hansen BD, Thomson A, *et al.* Evaluation of a digitally integrated accelerometer-based activity monitor for the measurement of activity in cats. *Vet Anaesth Analg* 2008;**35**:173–83.

66 Court MH, Greenblatt DJ. Molecular genetic basis for deficient acetaminophen glucuronidation by cats: UGRT1A6 is a pseudogene, and evidence for reduced diversity of expressed hepatic UGT1A isoforms. *Pharmacogenetics* 2000;**10**:355–69.

67 Gunew MN, Menrath VH, *et. al.* Long-term safety, efficacy and palatability of oral meloxicam at 0.01-0.03 mg/kg for treatment of osteoarthritic pain in cats. *J Feline Med Surg*, 2008 Jul; **10**(3):235–41.

68 Williams JT. The painless synergism of aspirin and opium. *Nature* 1997;**390**:557–9.

69 Lee A, Cooper MC, Craig JC, *et al.* Effects of nonsteroidal anti-inflammatory drugs on postoperative renal function in adults with normal renal function. *Cochrane Database of Systematic Reviews*, 2004. Issue 2: CD002765.

70 Omote K, Kawamata T, Nakayama Y, *et al.* Effects of a novel selective agonist for prostaglandin E receptor subtype EP4 on hyperalgesia and inflammation in a monarthritic model. *Anesthesiology* 2002;**97**:170–6.

71 Minami T, Nakano H, Kobayashi T, *et al.* Characterization of EP receptor subtypes

responsible for prostaglandin E2-induced pain responses by use of EP1 and EP3 receptor knockout mice. *Br J Pharmacol* 2001;**133**:438–44.

72 Clark P, Rowland SE, Denis D, *et al.* MF498 (N-{(4-(5,9-Diethoxy-6-oxo-6,8-dihydro-7H-pyrrolo(3,4-g) quinolin-7-yl)-3-m ethylbenzyl)sulfonyl)-2-(2-methoxyphenyl)acetamide), a selective E prostanoid receptor 4 antagonist, relieves joint inflammation and pain in rodent models of rheumatoid and osteoarthritis. *J Pharmacol Exp Ther.* 2008 May; **325**(2):425–34.

73 Chen Q, Muramoto K, Masaaki N, *et al.* A novel antagonist of the prostaglandin E(2) EP(4) receptor inhibits Th1 differentiation and Th17 expansion and is orally active in arthritis models. *Br J Pharmacol* 2010 May;**160**(2):292–310.

74 Southall MD and Vasko MR. Prostaglandin receptor subtypes, EP3C and EP4, mediate the prostaglandin E2-induced cAMP production and sensitization of sensory neurons. *J Biol Chem* 2001;**276**:16083–91.

75 Fitzgerald GA. Coxibs and cardiovascular disease. *N Engl J Med* 2004;**351**:1709–11.

76 Burkhardt D, Ghosh P. Laboratory evaluation of antiarthritic drugs as potential chondroprotective agents. *Sem Arthritis Rheumatol* 1987;**17**(2)Suppl 1:3–34.

77 Baici A, Salgram P, Fehr K, *et al.* Inhibition of human elastase from polymorphonuclear leukocytes by a glycosaminoglycan polysulfate (Arteparon). *Biochem Pharmacol* 1980;**29**:1723–7.

78 Stephens RW, Walton EA, Ghosh P, *et al.* A radioassay for proteolytic cleavage of isolated cartilage proteoglycan: inhibition of human leukocyte elastase and cathepsin G by anti-inflammatory drugs. *Arzneimittelforschung* 1980;**30**:2108–12.

79 Stancikova M, Trnavsky K, Keilova H. Effects of antirheumatic drugs on collagenolytic activity of cathepsin B1. *Biochem Pharmacol* 1977;**26**:2121–4.

80 Egg D. Effects of glycosaminoglycan polysulfate and two nonsteroidal anti-inflammatory drugs on prostaglandin E2 synthesis in Chinese hamster ovary cell cultures. *Pharm Res Commun* 1983;**15**:709–17.

81 Nishikawa H, Mori I, Umemoto J. Influences of sulfated glycosaminoglycans on biosynthesis of hyaluronic acid in rabbit knee synovia. *Arch Biochem Biophys* 1985;**240**:146–8.

82 Henrotin Y. Nutraceuticals in the management of osteoarthritis: an overview. *J Vet Pharmacol Ther* 2006;**29**(Suppl 1):201–10.

83 Cleland LG, James MN. Omega-3 fatty acids and synovitis in osteoarthritic knees. *J Nat Rev Rheumatol.* 2012;**8**:314–15.

84 Gruenwald J, Petzold E, Busch R, *et al.* Effect of glucosamine sulfate with or without omega-3 fatty acids in patients with osteoarthritis. *Adv Ther* 2009;**26**(9):858–71.

85 Hershman DL, Unger JM, Crew KD, *et al.* Randomized multicenter placebo-controlled trial of omega-3 fatty acids for the control of aromatase inhibitor-induced musculoskeltal pain. *J Clin Oncol* 2015;**33**:1910–17.

86 Hill CL, March LM, Aitken D, *et al.* Fish oil knee osteoarthritis: a randomized clinical trial of low dose versus high dose. *Ann Rheum Dis* 2016 Jan;**75**(1):23–9.

87 Knott L, Avery NC, Hollander AP, *et al.* Regulation of osteoarthritis by omega-3 polyunsaturated fatty acids in a naturally occurring model of disease. *Osteoarthr Cartilage* 2011;**19**:1150–7.

88 Lopez HL. Nutritional interventions to prevent and treat osteoarthritis. Part 1: focus on fatty acids and macronutrients *PMR.* 2012;**4**:S145–54.

89 Vandeweerd JM, Coisnon C, Clegg P, *et al.* Systemic review of efficacy of nutraceuticals to alleviate clinical signs of osteoarthritis. *J Vet Intern Med* 2012;**26**:448–56.

90 Wang Y, Wluka AE, Hodge AM, *et al.* Effect of fatty acids on bone marrow lesions and knee cartilage in healthy, middle-aged subjects without clinical knee osteoarthritis. *Osteoarthr Cartilage* 2008;**16**:579–83.

91 Wann AKT, Mistry J, Blain EJ, *et al.* Eicosapentaenoic acid and docosahexaenoic acid reduce interleukin-1β-mediated cartilage degradation. *Arthritis Res Ther* 2010;**12**(6):R207.

92 Fritsch DA, Allen TA, Dodd CE, *et al.* A multicenter study of the effect of dietary supplementation with fish oil omega-3 fatty acids on carprofen dosage in dogs with osteoarthritis. *J Am Vet Med Assoc* 2010;**236**:535–9.

93 Moreau M, Troncy E, del Castillo JRE, *et al.* Effects of feeding a high omega-3 fatty acids diet in dogs

with naturally occurring osteoarthritis. *J Anim Physiol and Anim Nutr (Berl)* 2013;**97**:830–7.

94 Roush JK, Dodd CE, Fritsch DA, *et al.* Multicenter veterinary practice assessment of the effects of omega-3 fatty acids on osteoarthritis in dogs. *J Am Vet Med Assoc* 2010;**236**:59–66.

95 Roush JK, Cross AR, Renberg WC, *et al.* Evaluation of the effects of dietary supplementation with fish oil omega-3 fatty acids on weight bearing in dogs with osteoarthritis. *J Am Vet Med Assoc* 2010;**236**:67–73.

96 Consumer Reports, January 2002, p. 19.

97 Animal Pharm Report, October (2005). www.animalpharmreports.com.

98 McAlindon TE, La Valley MP, Gulin JP, *et al.* Glucosamine and chondroitin for treatment of osteoarthritis: a systematic quality assessment and meta-analysis. *JAMA* 2000;**283**:1469–75.

99 Clegg DO, Reda DJ, Harris CL, *et al.* Glucosamine, chondroitin sulfate, and the two in combination for painful knee osteoarthritis. *NEJM* 2006;**354**(8):795–808.

100 Neil KM, Caron JP, Orth MW. The role of glucosamine and chondroitin sulfate in treatment for and prevention of osteoarthritis in animals. *JAVMA* 2006:**226**(7):1079–88.

101 Cwook JL, Anderson CC, Kreeger JM, *et.al.* Effects of human recombinant interleukin-1 beta on canine articular chondrocytes in three-dimensional culture. *AJVR* 2000;**61**:766.

102 Tung JT, Fenton JI, Arnold C, *et al.* Recombinant equine interleukin-1 beta induces putative mediator of articular cartilage degradation in equine chondrocytes. *Can J Vet Res* 2001;**66**:19–25.

103 Morris EA, Treadwell BV. Effect of interleukin 1 on articular cartilage from young and aged horses and comparison with metabolism of osteoarthritic cartilage. *AJVR* 1994;**55**:138–46.

104 Richardson DW, Dodge GR. Effects of interleukin-1 beta and tumor necrosis factor-alpha on expression of matrix-related genes by cultured equine articular chondrocytes. *AJVR* 2000;**61**:624–30.

105 MacDonald MH, Stover SM, Willits NH, *et al.* Regulation of matrix metabolism in equine cartilage explant cultures by interleukin 1. *AJVR* 1992;**53**:2278–85.

106 Platt D, Bayliss MT. An investigation of the proteoglycan metabolism of mature equine articular cartilage and its regulation by interleukin-1. *Equine Vet J* 1994;**26**:297–303.

107 Fenton JL, Chlebek-Brown KA, Caron JP, *et al.* Effect of glucosamine on interleukin-1-conditioned articular cartilage. *Equine Vet J (Suppl)* 2001;**34**:219–23.

108 Largo R, Alvarez-Soria MA, Diez-Ortego I, *et al.* Glucosamine inhibits IL-1 beta-induced NFkappaB activation in human osteoarthritic chondrocytes. *Osteoarthr Cartilage* 2003;**11**:290–8.

109 Bassleer C, Rovati L, Franchimont P. Stimulation of proteoglycan production by glucosamine sulfate in chondrocytes isolated from human osteoarthritic articular cartilage in vitro. *Osteoarthr Cartilage* 1998;**6**:427–34.

110 Orth MW, Peters TL, Hawkins JN. Inhibition of articular cartilage degradation by glucosamine-HCL and chondroitin sulphate. *Equine Vet J (Suppl)* 2002;**3**:224-9.

111 Bassleer C, Henrotin Y, Franchimont P. In vitro evaluation of drugs proposed as chondroprotective agents. *Int J Tissue React* 1992;**14**:231–41.

112 Fenton JL, Chlebek-Brown KA, Peters TL, *et al.* Glucosamine HCI reduces equine articular cartilage degradation in explant culture. *Osteoarthr Cartilage* 2000;**8**:258–65.

113 Byron CR, Orth MW, Venta PJ, *et al.* Influence of glucosamine on matrix metalloproteinase expression and activity in lipopolysaccharide-stimulated equine chondrocytes. *AJVR* 2003;**64**:666–71.

114 Dechant JE, Baxter GM, Frisbie DD, *et al.* Effects of glucosamine hydrochloride and chondroitin sulphate, alone and in combination, on normal and interleukin-1 conditioned equine articular cartilage explant metabolism. *Equine Vet J* 2005;**37**:227–31.

115 Sandy JD, Gamett D, Thompson V, *et al.* Chondrocyte-mediated catabolism of aggrecan: aggrecanse-dependent cleavage induced by interleukin-1 or retinoic acid can be inhibited by glucosamine. *Biochem J* 1998;**335**:59–66.

116 Shikhman AR, Kuhn K, Alaaeddine N, *et al.* N-acetylglucosamine prevents IL-1-beta-mediated activation of human chondrocytes. *J Immunol* 2001;**166**:5155–60.

117 Uebelhart D, Thonar DJ, Delmas PD, *et al.* Effects of oral chondroitin sulfate on the progression of knee osteoarthritis: a pilot study. *Osteoarthr Cartilage* 1998(suppl A):37–8.

118 Dodge CR, Jimenez SA. Glucosamine sulfate modulates the levels of aggrecan and matrix metalloproteinase-3 synthesized by cultured human osteoarthritis articular chondrocytes. *Osteoarthr Cartilage* 2003;**11**:424–32.

119 Gouze JN, Bianchi A, Becuwe P, *et al.* Glucosamine modulates IL-1-induced activation of rat chondrocytes at a receptor level, and by inhibiting the NF-kappa B pathway. *FEBS Lett* 2002;**510**:166–70.

120 Adebowale A, Du J, Liang Z, *et al.* The bioavailability and pharmacokinetics of glucosamine hydrochloride and low molecular weight chondroitin sulfate after single and multiple doses to beagle dogs. *Biopharm Drug Dispos* 2002;**23**:217–25.

121 Setnikar I, Palumbo R, Canali S, *et al.* Pharmacokinetics of glucosamine in man. *Arzneimittelforschung* 1993;**43**:1109–13.

122 McAlindon T. Why are clinical trials of glucosamine no longer uniformly positive? *Rheumatic Dis Clin N Am* 2003;**29**:789–801.

123 Grande D, O'Grady C, Garone E, *et al.* Chondroprotective and gene expression effects of nutritional supplements on articular cartilage. *Osteoarthr Cartilage* 2000;**8**(Suppl B):S34–5.

124 Rovati LC. Clinical development of glucosamine sulfate as selective drug in osteoarthritis. *Rheumatol Eur* 1997;**26**:70.

125 Dodge GR, Hawkins JF, Jimenez SA. Modulation of aggrecan, MMP1, and MMP3 productions by glucosamine sulfate in cultured human osteoarthritis articular chondrocytes. *Arthr Rheumatol* 1999;**42**S:253.

126 Piperno M, Reboul P, Hellio Le Graverand MP, *et al.* Glucosamine sulfate modulates dysregulated activities of human osteoarthritis chondrocytes in vitro. *Osteoarthr Cartilage* 2000;**8**:207–12.

127 Henrotin YE, Deberg MA, Crielaard JM, *et al.* Avocado/soybean unsaponifiables prevent the inhibitory effect of osteoarthritic subchondral osteoblasts on aggrecan and Type II collagen synthesis by chondrocytes. *J Rheumatol* 2006;**33**:1668–78.

128 Henrotin YE, Sanchez C, Deberg MA, *et al.* Avocado/soybean unsaponifiables increase aggrecan synthesis and reduce catabolic and proinflammatory mediator production by human osteoarthritic chondrocytes. *J Rheumatol* 2003;**30**:1825–34.

129 Boileau C, Martel-Pelletier J, Caron J, *et al.* Protective effects of total fraction of avocado/soybean unsaponifiables on the structural changes in experimental dog osteoarthritis: inhibition of nitric oxide synthase and matrix metalloproteinase-13. *Arthr Res Therapy* 2009;**11**:1–9.

130 Au RY, Al-Tallinn TK, Au AY, *et al.* Avocado soybean unsaponifiables (ASU) suppress TNF-α, IL-1β, COX-2, iNOS gene expression, and prostaglandin E2 and nitric oxide production in articular chondrocytes and monocyte/macrophages. *Osteoarthr Cartilage* 2007;**15**:1249–55.

131 Heineken LF, Grzanna MW, Au AY, *et al.* Inhibition of cyclooxygenase-2 expression and prostaglandin E2 production in chondrocytes by avocado soybean unsaponifiables and epigallocatechin gallate. *Osteoarthr Cartilage* 2010;**18**:220–7.

132 Grzanna MW, Ownby SL, Heineken LF, *et al.* Inhibition of cytokine expression and prostaglandin E2 production in monocyte/macrophage-like cells by avocado/soybean unsaponifiables and chondroitin sulfate. *J Comp Integ Med* 2010;**7**:1–16.

133 Haqqi TM, Anthony DD, Gupta S, , *et al.* Prevention of collagen-induced arthritis in mice by a polyphenolic fraction from green tea. *Proc Natl Acad Sci USA* 1999;**96**(8):4524–9.

134 Morinobu A, Biao W, Tanaka S, *et al.* Epigallocatechin-3-gallate suppresses osteoclast differentiation and ameliorates experimental arthritis in mice. *Arthritis Rheum* 2008;**58**(7):2012–18.

135 Heinecke LF, Grzanna MW, Au AY, *et al.* Inhibition of cyclooxygenase-2 expression and prostaglandin E2 production in chondrocytes by avocado soybean unsaponifiables and epigallocatechin gallate. *Osteoarthr Cartilage* 2010 Feb. **18**(2):220–7.

136 Frondoza CG, Heinecke LF, Grzanna MW, *et al.* 2012

OARSI World Congress on Osteoarthritis; poster #475.

137 Data on file: Nutramax Laboratories Veterinary Sciences, Inc. 2012.

138 Singh S, Aggarwal BB. Activation of transcription factor NFkB is suppressed by curcumin (diferuloylmethane). *J Biol Chem* 1995;**270**:2495–500.

139 Surh YJ, Chun KS, Cha HH, *et al*. Molecular mechanism underlying chemopreventive activities of anti-inflammatory phytochemicals: down regulation of COX-2 and iNOS through suppression of NF-κB activation. *Mutat Res* 2001; **480–481**:243–68.

140 Chattopadhyay I, Biswas K, Bandyopadhyay U, *et al*. Turmeric and curcumin: Biological actions and medicinal applications. *Curr Sci* **87**.

141 Clutterbuck AL, Allaway D, Harris P, *et al*. Curcumin reduces prostaglandin E2, matrix metalloproteinase-3 and proteoglycan release in the secretome of interleukin 1β-treated articular cartilage. [v2; ref status: indexed, http://f1000r. es/1ks] F1000Research 2013, 2:147 (doi: 10.12688/ f1000research.2-147.v2.

142 Reddy CM, Bhat VB, Kiranmai G, *et al*. Selective inhibition of cyclooxygenase-2 by C-phycocyanin, a biliprotein from *Spirulina platensis*. *Biochem Biophys Res Comm* 2000;**277**:599–603.

143 Romay C, Ledón N, González R. Further studies on anti-inflammatory activity of phycocyanin in some animal models of inflammation. *Inflamm Res* 1998;**47**:334–8.

144 Cherng S, Cheng S, Tarn A, *et al*. Anti-inflammatory activity of c-phycocyanin in lipopolysaccharide-stimulated RAW 264.7 macrophages. *Life Sci* 2007;**81**:1431–5.

145 CDC Guideline for Prescribing Opiates for Chronic Pain – United States, 2016. Recommendations and Reports March 18, 2016;**65**(1):1–49.

146 May TJ. Crotalin. An improved method for its administration. *Boston Med Surg J* 1910;**162**:46–7.

147 Jenkins CL, Pendleton AS. Crotalin in epilepsy. *JAMA* 1914;**63**(20):1749–50.

148 Gosset. Cobra venom in cancer. *Lancet (Paris)*. 1933;Apr 15:826.

149 Gomes A, Bhattacharya S, Chakraborty M, *et. al*. Anti-arthritic activity of Indian monocellate cobra (*Naja kaouthia*) venom on adjuvant induced arthritis. *Toxicon* 2010 Feb-Mar;**55**(2-3):670–3.

150 Macht DI. Experimental and clinical study of cobra venom as an analgesic. *Proc Natl Acad Sci USA* 1936;**22**(1):61–71.

151 Zang HL, Han R, Gu ZL, *et al*. A short-chain a-neurotoxin from *Naja naja atra* produces potent cholinergic-dependent analgesia. *Neurosci Bull* 2006;**22**(2):103–9.

152 Chen ZX, Zang HL, Gu ZL, *et al*. A long-form α-neurotoxin from cobra venom produces potent opioid-independent analgesia. *Acta Pharmacol Sin* 2006;**27**(4):402–8.

153 Liu YL, Lin HM, Zou R, *et al*. Suppression of complete Freund's adjuvant-induced adjuvant arthritis by cobratoxin. *Acta Pharmacol Sin* 2009;**30**(2):219–27.

154 Koh DC, Armugam A, Jeyaseelan K. Snake venom components and their applications in biomedicine. *Cell Mol Life Sci* 2006;**63**(24):3030–41.

155 Damaj MI, Fei-Yin M, Dukat M, *et al*. Antinociceptive responses to nicotinic acetylcholine receptor ligands after systemic and intrathecal administration in mice. *J Pharmacol Exp Ther* 1998;**284**(3):1058–65.

156 Catassi A, Paleari L, Servent D, *et al*. Targeting alpha7-nicotinic receptor for the treatment of pleural mesothelioma. *Eur J Cancer* 2008;**44**(15):2296–311.

157 Reid PF. Cobra venom: a review of the old alternative to opiate analgesia. *Altern Ther Health Med* 2011;**17**(1):58–71.

158 Wang X, Wang F, Hu ZD. Effect of new cobratoxin on postoperative analgesia. *J Snake* 1999;**11**(1):19–20.

159 Adebowale AO, Cox DS, Liang Z, *et al*. Analysis of glucosamine and chondroitin sulfate content in marketed products and the Caco-2 permeability of chondroitin sulfate raw materials. *J Am Nutrit Assoc* 2000;**3**:37–44.

160 Russell AS, Aghazadeh-Habashi A, Jamali F. Active ingredient consistency of commercially available glucosamine sulfate products. *J Rheumatol* 2002;**29**:2407–9.

161 FDA. Available at: www.fda.gov//ohrms/dockets/ dailys/04/oct04/101304/04p-0060/pdn0001-yoc. htm as accessed 27 April 2005.

162 Oke SL. Indications and contraindications for the

use of orally administered joint health products in dogs and cats. *JAVMA* 2009;**234**:1393–7.

163 McQuay HJ, Moore A. NSAIDs and coxibs: clinical use. In: McMahon SB, Koltzenburg M (eds). *Wall and Melzack's Textbook of Pain,* edn 5. Elsevier Churchill Livingston, Philadelphia, 2006, pp. 471–80.

164 Bianchi M, Broggini M, Balzarini P, *et al.* Effects of tramadol on synovial fluid concentrations of substance P and interleukin-6 in patients with knee osteoarthritis: comparison with paracetamol. *Int Immunopharm* 2003;**3**(13–14):1901–8.

165 American College of Rheumatology Subcommittee on Osteoarthritis. Recommendations for the medical management of osteoarthritis of the hip and knee. *Arthritis Rheumatol* 2000;**43**:1905–15.

166 American Medical Directors' Association. *Chronic Pain Management in the Long-term Care Setting: Clinical Practice Guideline.* American Medical Directors' Association, Baltimore, 1999, p. i–32.

167 Cepeda MS, Camargo F, Zea C, *et al.* Tramadol for osteoarthritis. *Cochrane Database of Systematic Reviews* 2006, Issue 3. Art. No: CD005522. DOI:10.1002/14651858.CD005522.pub2

168 Torring ML, Riis A, Christensen S, *et al.* Perforated peptic ulcer and short-term mortality among tramadol users. *British J Clin Pharm* 2007;**65**:565–72.

169 Garcia-Hernandez L, Deciga-Campos M, Guevara-Lopez U, *et al.* Co-administration of rofecoxib and tramadol results in additive or sub-additive interaction during arthritic nociception in rat. *Pharm Bio Behav* 2007;**87**:331–40.

170 Abate, M, Salini, V. *Hyaluronic Acid in the Treatment of Osteoarthritis: What is New, Osteoarthritis - Diagnosis, Treatment and Surgery*, Prof. Qian Chen (ed.), inTech, Italy, 2012, pp. 102–114. ISBN 978-953-51-0168-0.

171 Wang CT, Lin J, Chang CJ, *et al.* Therapeutic effects of hyaluronic acid on osteoarthritis of the knee. A met-analysis of randomized controlled trials. *J Bone Joint Surg Am* 2004;Mar **86**-A(3):538–45.

172 Marshall KW. Intra-articular hyaluronan therapy. *Curr Opin Rheumatol* 2000 Sep;**12**(5):468–74.

173 Takahashi K, Hashimoto S, Kubo T, *et al.* Haluronan suppressed nitric oxide production

in the meniscus and synovium of rabbit osteoarthritis model. *J Orthop Res* 2001 May; **19**(3):500–3.

174 Gigante A, Callegari L. The role of intra-articular hyaluronan (Sinovial) in the treatment of osteoarthritis. *Rheumatol Int* 2011;**31**(4): 427–44.

175 Pozo MA, Balazs EA, Belmonte C. Reduction of sensory responses to passive movements of inflamed knee joints by hylan, a hyaluronan derivative. *Exp Brain Res* 1997 Aug;**116**(1):3–9.

176 Kumahashi N, Naitou K, Nishi H, *et al.* Correlation of changes in pain intensity with synovial fluid adenosine triphosphate levels after treatment of patients with osteoarthritis of the knee with high-molecular-weight hyaluronic acid. *Knee* 2011;**18**(3):160–4.

177 Wang CT, Lin J, Chang CJ, *et al.* Therapeutic effects of hyaluronic acid on osteoarthritis of the knee. A meta-analysis of randomized controlled trials. *J Bone Joint Surg Am* Mar 2004;**86**-A(3):538–45.

178 Balogh L, Polyak A, Mathe D, *et al.* Absorption, uptake and tissue affinity of high-molecular-weight hyaluronan after oral administration in rats and dogs. *J Agric Food Chem* 2008;**56**:10582–93.

179 Liu NF. Trafficking of hyaluronan in the interstitium and its possible implications. *Lymphology* 2004;**37**:6–14.

180 Campo GM, Avenoso A, D'Ascola A, *et al.* Hyaluronan differently modulates TLR-4 and the inflammatory response in mouse chondrocytes. *Biofactors* 2012;**38**: 69–76.

181 Frizziero L, Govoni E, Bacchini P. Intra-articular hyaluronic acid in the treatment of osteoarthritis of the knee: clinical and morphological study. *Clin Exp Rheumatol* 1998;**16**:441–9.

182 World Health Organization. *WHO Traditional Medicine Strategy 2002–2005.* World Health Organization, Geneva, 2002.

183 Bache F. Cases illustrative of the remedial effects of acupuncture. *N Am Med Surg J* 1826;**2**:311–21.

184 Skarda RT, Glowaski M. Acupuncture. In: Tranquilli WJ, Thurman JC, Grimm KA (eds). *Lumb and Jones' Veterinary Anesthesia and Analgesia*, edn 4. Blackwell, Ames, IA, 2007, pp. 683–97.

185 Ma Y, Cho ZH (eds). *Biomedical Acupuncture for Pain Management: an Integrative Approach.* Elsevier, St. Louis, 2005.

186 Helms JM. *Acupuncture Energetics: A Clinical*

Approach for Physicians. Medical Acupuncture Publishers, Berkeley, CA, 1997.

187 Pomeranz B, Chiu D. Naloxone blockade of acupuncture analgesia. Endorphin implicated. *Life Sci* 1976;**19**:1757–62.

188 Lee A, Done ML. The use of nonpharmacologic techniques to prevent postoperative nausea and vomiting. A meta-analysis. *Anesth Analg* 1999;**88**:1362–9.

189 American Cancer Society. *American Cancer Society's Guide to Complementary and Alternative Cancer Methods*. American Cancer Society, Atlanta, 2000.

190 Kapatkin AS, Tomasic M, Beech J, *et al.* Effects of electrostimulated acupuncture on ground reaction forces and pain scores in dogs with chronic elbow joint arthritis. *JAVMA* 2006;**228**(9):1350–4.

191 Benito MJ, Veale DJ, FitzGerald O, *et al.* Synovial tissue inflammation in early and late osteoarthritis. *Ann Rheum Dis* 2005;**64**:1263–7.

192 Sokolove J, Lepus CM. Role of inflammation in the pathogenesis of osteoarthritis: latest findings and interpretations. *Ther Adv Musculoskelet Dis* 2013;**5**:77–94.

193 Scanzello CR, Umoh E, Pessler F, *et al.* Local cytokine profiles in knee osteoarthritis: elevated synovial fluid interleukin-15 differentiates early from end-stage disease. *Osteoarthr Cartilage* 2009;**17**:1040–8.

194 Bondeson J, Wainwright SD, Lauder S, *et al.* The role of synovial macrophages and macrophage-produced cytokines in driving aggrecanases, matrix metalloproteinases, and other destructive and inflammatory responses in osteoarthritis. *Arthritis Res Ther* 2006;**8**:R187.

195 de Lange-Brokaar BJ, Ioan-Facsinay A, van Osch GJ, *et al.* Synovial inflammation, immune cells and their cytokines in osteoarthritis: a review. *Osteoarthr Cartilage* 2012;**12**:1484–99.

196 Poole AR. An introduction to the pathophysiology of osteoarthritis. *Front Biosci* 1999;**4**:D662–70.

197 McDougall JJ. Arthritis and pain: Neurogenic origin of joint pain. *Arthritis Res Ther* 2006;**8**:220.

198 Delbarre F, Cayla J, Menkes C, *et al.* [Synoviorthesis with radioisotopes]. *Presse Med* 1968;**76**:1045–50.

199 Kampen WU, Voth M, Pinkert J, *et al.* Therapeutic status of radiosynoviorthesis of the knee with yttrium [90Y] colloid in rheumatoid arthritis and related indications. *Rheumatology* 2007;**46**:16–24.

200 Karavida N, Notopoulos A. Radiation synovectomy: an effective alternative treatment for inflamed small joints. *Hippokratia* 2010;**14**:22–7.

201 Klett R, Lange U, Haas H, *et al.* Radiosynoviorthesis of medium-sized joints with rhenium-186-sulfide colloid: a review of the literature. *Rheumatology* 2007;**46**:1531–7.

202 Modder G. Rheumatoid and related joint diseases. In: *Radiosynoviorthesis. Involvement of Nuclear Medicine in Rheumatolopgy and Orthopaedics*. Warlich Druck Verlagsges, MbH, Meckenheim, Germany; 1995, pp. 13–23.

203 Rodriguez-Merchan EC, Wiedel JD. General principles and indications of synoviorthesis (medical synovectomy) in haemophilia. *Haemophilia* 2001;**7** (Suppl2):6–10.

204 Silva M, Luck JV Jr, Llinas A. Chronic hemophilic synovitis: The role of radiosynovectomy. *Treatment Hemophilia* 2004;**33**:1–10.

205 Yarbrough TB, Lee MR, Hornof WJ, *et al.* Samarium 153-labeled hydroxyapatite microspheres for radiation synovectomy in the horse: a study of the biokinetics, dosimetry, clinical, and morphologic response in normal metacarpophalangeal and metatarsophalangeal joints. *Vet Surg* 2000;**29**:191–9.

206 Stevenson N, Lattimer J, Selting K, *et al.* Abstract S6-03: Homogenous Sn-117m colloid - A novel radiosynovectomy agent. *World J Nucl Med* 2015;**14**(Suppl 1):S15–68.

207 Stevenson NR, St. George G, Simon J, *et al.* Methods of producing high specific activity Sn-117m with commercial cyclotrons. *J Radioanal Nucl Chem* 2015;**305**:99–108.

208 Atkins HL, Mausner LF, Srivastava SC, *et al.* Tin-117m(4+)-DTPA for palliation of pain from osseous metastases: a pilot study. *J Nucl Med* 1995;**36**:725–9.

209 Krishnamurthy GT, Swailem FM, Srivastava SC, *et al.* Tin-117m(4+)DTPA: pharmacokinetics and imaging characteristics in patients with metastatic bone pain. *J Nucl Med* 1997;**38**:230–7.

210 Srivastava SC, Atkins HL, Krishnamurthy GT, *et al.* Treatment of metastatic bone pain with tin-117m Stannic diethylenetriaminepentaacetic acid: a phase I/II clinical study. *Clin Cancer Res* 1998;**4**:61–68.

211 Srivastava SC. The role of electron-emitting

radiopharmaceuticals in the palliative treatment of metastatic bone pain and for radiosynovectomy: applications of conversion electron emitter Tin-117m. *Brazilian Arch Biol Technol* 2007;**50**:49–62.

212 LaRue SM, Custis JT. Advances in veterinary radiation therapy: targeting tumors and improving patient comfort. *Vet Clin North Am (SAP)* 2014;**44**:909–23.

213 Mäkelä OT, Lammi MJ, Uusitalo H, *et al.* Effect of radiosynovectomy with holmium-166 ferric hydroxide macroaggregate on adult equine cartilage. *J Rheumatol* 2004;**31**:321–8.

214 Mäkelä O, Sukura A, Penttilä P, *et al.* Radiation synovectomy with holmium-166 ferric hydroxide macroaggregate in equine metacarpophalangeal and metatarsophalangeal joints. *Vet Surg* 2003;**32**:402–9.

215 Vallance SA, Lumsden JM, Begg AP, *et al.* Idiopathic haemarthrosis in eight horses. *Aust Vet J* 2012;**90**:214–20.

216 Hugenberg ST, Myers SL, Brandt KD. Suppression of glycosaminoglycan synthesis by articular cartilage, but not of hyaluronic acid synthesis by synovium, after exposure to radiation. *Arthritis Rheum* 1989;**32**:468–74.

217 Myers SL, Slowman SD, Brandt KD. Radiation synovectomy stumlates glycosaminoglycan synthesis by normal articular cartilage. *J Lab Clin Med* 1989;**114**:27–35.

218 Polyak A, Das t, Chakraborty S, *et al.* Thulium-170-labeled microparticles for local radiotherapy: preliminary studies. *Cancer Biother Radiopharm* 2014;**29**:330–8.

219 Kunst CM, Pease AP, Nelson NC, *et al.* Computed tomographic identification of dysplasia and progression of osteoarthritis in dog elbows previously assigned OFA grades 0 and 1. *Vet Radiol Ultrasound* 2014;**55**:511–20.

220 Cook RJ, Sackett DL. The number needed to treat: a clinically useful measure of treatment effect. *BMJ* 1995;**310**:452–4.

221 Edwards JE, McQuay HJ, Moore RA. Combination analgesic efficacy: individual patient data meta-analysis of single-dose oral tramadol plus acetaminophen in acute postoperative pain. *J Pain Symptom Manage* 2002;**23**:121–30.

222 Muller M, Kersten S. Nutrigenomics: goals and strategies. *Nature Rev* 2003;**4**:315–22.

223 Vester BM, Swanson K. Nutrient-gene interactions: application to pet nutrition and health. *Vet Focus* 2007;**17**:25–32.

224 Eisele I, Wood IS, German AJ, *et al.* Adipokine gene expression in dog adipose tissues and dog white adipocytes differentiated in primary culture. *Horm Metabol Res* 2005;**37**:474–81.

225 Trayhurn P, Wood IS. Adipokines: inflammation and the pleiotropic role of white adipose tissue. *Br J Nutrition* 2004;**92**:347–55.

226 Wander RC, Hall JA, Gradin JL, *et al.* The ratio of dietary (n-6) to (n-3) fatty acids influences immune system function, eicosanoid metabolism, lipid peroxidation, and vitamin E status in aged dogs. *J Nutr* 1997;**127**:1198–205.

227 Schwab JM, Serhan CN. Lipoxins and new lipid mediators in the resolution of inflammation. *Curr Opin Pharmacol* 2006;**6**:414–20.

228 Serhan CN. Novel omega-3-derived local mediators in anti-inflammation and resolution. *Pharmaco Ther* 2005;**105**:7–21.

229 Clinician's Update™, Supplement to NAVC Clinician's Brief®. April 2005.

Chapter 4

Physical Rehabilitation in the Treatment of Osteoarthritis

INTRODUCTION

Historically, arthritis management has been focused on pharmacologic intervention, i.e. managing the pain. While pain management is, unquestionably, the primary focus of managing osteoarthritis (OA), there are other modalities that appear to be efficacious in treating OA pain. Canine physiotherapy/rehabilitation is a discipline that encompasses the application of physical therapy techniques to dogs whose comfort and function have been compromised. Commonly used techniques include cryotherapy, thermotherapy, physical rehabilitation and therapeutic exercises, transcutaneous electrical nerve stimulation (TENS), low-level laser, magnets, and extracorporeal shock wave treatment. Acute response to treatment is most pronounced, yet long-lasting results have been acknowledged for some modalities.

The very term 'physical rehabilitation' suggests previous trauma or significant compromise, yet the overall goal of physiotherapy/rehabilitation is to restore, maintain, and promote optimal function, optimal fitness, wellness, and quality of life as they relate to movement disorders and health. Techniques used in physical rehabilitation are broad-reaching; as may be appropriate for the diversification of patients' debilitations. Some modalities are as simplistic as leash walking, which can easily be administered by the pet owner. On the other hand, some modalities are complex, sophisticated techniques, requiring administration by professional personnel sufficiently trained with inclusive knowledge of risks and precautions for these modalities.

ENVIRONMENTAL MODIFICATION

It is difficult to overstate the positive difference that simple environmental changes can make for the maladaptive pain patient. Yet, this is one area that is easy to overlook because it does not involve as much 'hard science' as choosing a pharmacologic regimen or calculating an appropriate nutritional profile. With a few simple questions it is fairly straightforward to determine if the rehabilitation patient will benefit from environmental modification. It does mean taking the initiative to gather information about the home, such as floor surfaces, stairs, placement of food and water dishes, type of bedding, location of bedding, and so on.

One of the simplest environmental modifications that can have a positive effect on the chronically painful rehabilitation patient is to protect the dog from slippery floor surfaces. Aging patients, particularly those with OA, experience a loss of proprioceptive function in joint receptors compared with younger patients, particularly in the presence of OA. Non-skid area rugs, flooring used in children's play areas, and rubber-backed mats are some examples of ways a dog owner can make the home more comfortable for the painful patient.

Raising food and water dishes to between elbow and shoulder height makes for more comfortable meal times. Be sure the dog is able to stand on a non-skid surface while eating and drinking. Have the client explore the home for potential 'problem spots'. Steps in and out of the house, patio stones, and garage floors can create unintentional challenges for the painful dog. Ramps are recommended for getting into and out of vehicles. Likewise, have the client consider ramps or steps if the dog is used to getting onto and off furniture. It may be best to use child restraint gates at the top and bottom of staircases to prevent unsupervised access. Memory foam or 'egg-shell' foam may make for a more comfortable sleeping surface for the painful dog. Assistive devices like slings and 'walking wheelchairs' can sustain mobility during the initiation of appropriate multimodal pain management strategies. Finally, it is best for the dog to receive moderate exercise every day than to do excessive exercise on the weekend, requiring the rest of the week to recover.

PAIN PATHOPHYSIOLOGY RELATED TO PHYSICAL REHABILITATION

In response to injury, specialized nerve endings (nociceptors) are activated which transmit nerve signals through the spinal cord to the brain, where the sensations of pain are cognitively recognized. Almost simultaneously, neurotransmitters initiate a spinal reflex that increases muscle motor activity and tonicity at the site of injury, leading to a reflexive muscle contraction. If persistent, the increase in muscle tone can cause painful muscle spasms, which may lead to further tissue damage due to decreased blood flow and oxygen (hypoxia) in the surrounding tissues. This precipitates cyclic pain, and the injury process is called the pain–spasm–pain cycle (**4.1**). To reduce the pain or unpleasant sensation, this cycle must be broken or interrupted.

Many of the physical modalities used for the management of OA in veterinary patients are derived from use in human OA patients. However, there is great variability in the recommended implementation of various modalities. In 2007, the Osteoarthritis Research Society International Treatment Guidelines Committee reported on a critical appraisal of published guidelines and systematic review of recent evidence for relevant therapies for the management of hip and knee OA in humans[1]. Among the 1462 published guidelines reviewed that met the inclusion/exclusion criteria, 23 guidelines were developed for the treatment of hip and/or knee OA. Twenty of 51 modalities of therapy were universally recommended by these guidelines.

Optimal management of patients with OA hip or knee requires a combination of nonpharmacologic and pharmacologic modalities of therapy. Recommendations cover the use of 12 nonpharmacologic modalities: education and self-management, regular telephone contact, referral to a physical therapist, aerobic, muscle strengthening, and water-based exercises, weight reduction, walking aids, knee braces, footwear and insoles, thermal modalities, TENS, and acupuncture.

Eight recommendations cover pharmacologic modalities of treatment including acetaminophen, cyclo-oxygenase (COX)-2 nonselective and selective oral nonsteroidal anti-inflammatory drugs (NSAIDs), topical NSAIDs and capsaicin, intra-articular injections of corticosteroids and hyaluronates, glucosamine and/or chondroitin sulphate for symptom relief; glucosamine sulphate, chondroitin sulphate, and diacerein for possible structure-modifying effects, and the use of opioid analgesics for the treatment of refractory pain. There are recommendations covering five surgical modalities: total joint replacements, uni-compartmental knee replacement, osteotomy, and joint preserving surgical procedures; joint lavage and arthroscopic debridement in knee OA, and joint fusion as a salvage procedure when joint replacement has failed.

Thermoreceptors, special temperature-sensitive nerve endings, which are activated by changes in skin temperature, initiate nerve signals that block nociception within the spinal cord (**4.2**). Another type of specialized nerve ending, called proprioceptors, detect physical changes in tissue pressure and movement. Proprioceptor activity can also inhibit the transmission of nociception signals to the brain.

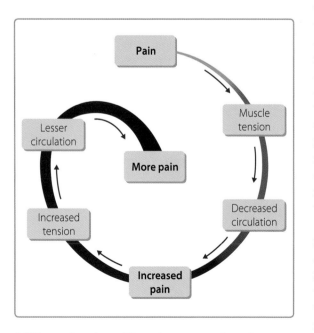

4.1 The cyclic nature of the pain–spasm–pain cycle.

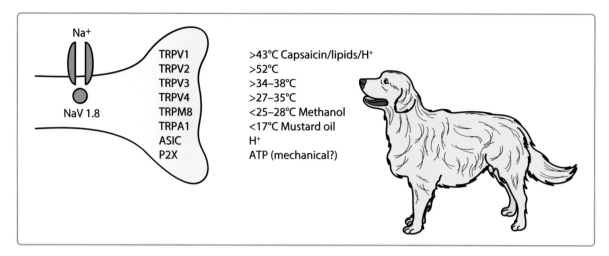

Na+		
	TRPV1	>43°C Capsaicin/lipids/H+
	TRPV2	>52°C
	TRPV3	>34–38°C
	TRPV4	>27–35°C
NaV 1.8	TRPM8	<25–28°C Methanol
	TRPA1	<17°C Mustard oil
	ASIC	H+
	P2X	ATP (mechanical?)

4.2 Thermoreceptors, such as the family of transient receptor potential (e.g. transient receptor potential vanilloid V1, TRPV1) are activated at different temperature ranges. ATP: adenosine triphosphate.

Activity of these receptors within the spinal cord reduces muscle tone, relaxes painful muscles, and enhances tissue blood flow (**4.3**). Topical hot and cold modalities have been used since antiquity for the treatment of musculoskeletal injuries; however, only recently has there been an understanding of the complexity of their physiologic actions. Although cold and hot treatment modalities both decrease pain and muscle spasm, they have opposite effects on tissue metabolism, blood flow, inflammation, edema, and connective tissue extensibility (*Table 4.1*).

CRYOTHERAPY

Cryotherapy decreases tissue blood flow by causing vasoconstriction, and reduces tissue metabolism, oxygen utilization, and muscle spasm[2–4]. As a result of the decreased circulation, cold penetrates deeper and lasts longer than heat. At joint temperatures of 30°C (86°F) or lower, the activity of cartilage degrading enzymes, including collagenase, elastase, hyaluronidase, and protease is inhibited[5]. Cold raises the activation threshold of tissue nociceptors, increases the duration of the refractory period, and reduces nerve conduction velocity of pain nerves. The result is a local anesthetic effect called cold-induced neuropraxia[6,7].

Cryotherapy works by both neurologic and vascular mechanisms to yield effects locally and at the level of the spinal cord. Topical cold treatment decreases the temperature of the skin and underlying tissues to a depth of 1–3 cm, decreasing the activation threshold of tissue nociceptors and the conduction velocity of pain nerve signals[8]. Various methods such as ice packs[9], ice towels, ice massage[10], gel packs, refrigerant gases, and inflatable splints can be used. Cold is used to reduce the recovery time as part of the rehabilitation program both

Table 4.1 Effects of temperature on physiologic actions

	Cold	Heat
Pain	▼	▼
Spasm	▼	▼
Metabolism	▼	▲
Blood flow	▼	▲
Inflammation	▼	▲
Edema	▼	▲
Extensibility	▼	▲

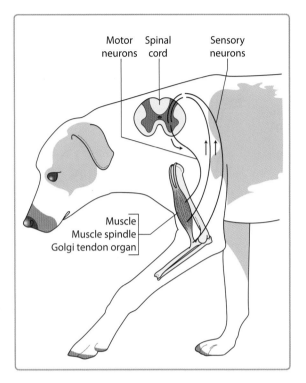

Motor neurons **Spinal cord** **Sensory neurons**

Muscle
Muscle spindle
Golgi tendon organ

4.3 Skeletal muscle hosts the neuromuscular spindles. There are more of these in muscles of the limbs than elsewhere. These proprioceptors are responsible for sending information back to the brain that determines the increase or decrease in muscle tension, which is determined by the lengthening or stretching of individual fibers. This relays information regarding the rate of muscle contraction as well as the speed of muscle contraction. The endings of the sensory neurons spiral around particular muscle fibers in order to sense the changes in each individual muscle fiber, which in turn permits them to discern this information.

after acute injuries and in the treatment of chronic injuries.

A bone scanning study[11] demonstrated that the application of an ice wrap to one (human) knee for 20 minutes decreased arterial blood flow by 38%, soft tissue blood flow by 26%, and bone uptake (which reflects changes in bone blood flow and metabolism) by 19%. From a Cochrane Database of Systematic Reviews, authors reviewed three randomized controlled trials, involving 179 human patients[12]. In one trial, administration of 20 minutes of ice massage, 5 day per week, for

3 weeks, compared to control demonstrated a clinically important benefit for knee OA on increasing quadriceps strength (20% relative difference). There was also a statistically significant improvement in knee flexion range of motion (ROM) and functional status. Ice massage compared to control had a statistically beneficial effect on ROM, function, and knee strength. Additionally cold packs were shown to decrease swelling. One study has shown that ice massage reduces the appearance of plasma creatine kinase following muscle damage[13].

Cold compression therapy has been shown to decrease immediate postoperative pain and lameness and increase range of motion in the stifle joint of dogs after tibial plateau leveling osteotomy[14].

The different types of cryotherapy are presented in *Table 4.2*.

Precautions and contraindications
Frostbite is a potential complication of cryotherapy, therefore signs of frostbite should be monitored throughout and following treatment. Caution should also be taken when applying cryotherapy in the vicinity of superficial nerves and areas of decreased perfusion[21–24]. One might intuitively think that the animal's hair coat acts as an insulating barrier to the application of cold, but this may not be the case[25].

THERMOTHERAPY

Thermotherapy is the therapeutic application of any substance to the body that adds heat resulting in increased tissue temperature. Heat therapy can be either superficial (up to approximately 2 cm) or deep (3 cm or more) and, like cryotherapy, it provides analgesia and decreased muscle tonicity. In contrast to cryotherapy, thermotherapy increases tissue temperature, blood flow, metabolism, and connective tissue extensibility. Heat is carried away by circulation more rapidly than cold, but nevertheless, both heat and cold relieve pain and muscle spasm[16]. Heat causes general relaxation of painful muscle spasms, and may inhibit motor neurons, helping to break the pain–spasm–pain cycle. Heat therapy is delivered in three modalities: radiant (infrared lamp), conduction (hot pack), and convection (whirlpool).

Table 4.2 Applications of cryotherapy

Modality	Comments
Ice packs	Covering ice packs with a single layer of wet towel can enhance heat exchange Apply ice packs for up to 10–20 min 15 min on : 60 min off (empirical) Ice packs can consist of crushed ice or a bag of 'frozen peas' can be substituted 1/3 part isopropyl alcohol with 2/3 part water placed in a resealable plastic bag can be kept in a freezer
Commercially available cold packs	Often made of silica gel in plastic or canvas covers Most are less efficient than ice[15]
Iced towels	Soaked in ice-water slush Towels warm quickly, therefore alternate a two-towel 'exchange'
Ice wrap bandages	Often marketed for horses and humans May be maintained in the refrigerator
Ice gels	Variable retention of cold (material dependent)
Ice massage	'Popsicle'-like ice Rubbed over small area provides massage while cooling Pressure from massage stimulates mechanoreceptors more than other forms of cryotherapy Applied parallel to muscle fibers, for 5–10 min or until the affected area is erythematous and numb
Cold/compression	As with a circulating coolant boot Efficacy established in horses[16]
Cold bath	Immersion of body part in cool or icy 'slush' water Cool, cold, or very cold bath[17]
Vapocoolant sprays	Highly volatile liquids that cause evaporative cooling
Contrast baths	Alternating immersion in warm and cold water 'Vascular exercise' producing vasodilation and vasoconstriction Support for efficacy appears anecdotal[18] Research has demonstrated the superior effects of continuous cryotherapy and thermotherapy in the treatment of pain as opposed to intermittent treatment[19,20]

A 1°C increase in tissue temperature is associated with a 10–15% increase in local tissue metabolism[26]. Resultant increased blood flow facilitates tissue healing by supplying proteins, nutrients, and oxygen to the site of injury. Conductive topical heat treatment of the knees of healthy human subjects increased popliteal artery blood flow by 29%, 94%, and 200% after 35 minutes of treatment with heating pad temperatures of 38°C, 40°C, and 43°C, respectively[27]. Erasala *et al.* demonstrated that deep tissue blood flow was found to increase by 27%, 77%, and 144% in the trapezius muscle of healthy human volunteers with heating pad treatments, resulting in skin temperature increases to 38°C, 40°C, and 42°C, respectively[28]. Further, functional brain imaging has revealed that non-noxious skin warming increases activation of the thalamus and posterior insula of the brain, contributing to pain relief[29]. There are no scientific data supporting the contention that moist heat is therapeutically superior to dry heat.

Nadler *et al.* showed that heat, topically applied to the skin, was superior to both acetaminophen and ibuprofen in the treatment of acute lower back pain for all therapeutic measurements, including pain relief, muscle stiffness, lateral trunk flexibility, and disability[30]. Two days after treatment was discontinued, extended pain relief was significantly greater for the heat wrap than for either acetaminophen or ibuprofen.

In a human rheumatoid arthritis model, investigators demonstrated that fibroblast-like synoviocytes exposed to hyperthermia showed reductions in interleuking (IL)-1α-induced prostaglandin E2 release, suppression of activation of the adhesion molecules vascular cell adhesion molecule 1 (VCAM-1), intercellular cell adhesion molecule 1 (ICAM-1), the cytokines tumor necrosis factor (TNFα), IL-1α, IL-8, as well as COX-2 protein synthesis[31]. These investigators demonstrated by Western blot that fibroblast-like synoviocytes exposed to hyperthermia were suppressed in the phosphorylation and subsequent degradation of IkBα (inhibitor of kappa B), thereby retaining the nuclear factor kappa-light-chain-enhancer of activated B cell (NF-kB) complex in the cell cytoplasm; the clinical relevance being that there was suppressed phosphorylation and decreased production of inflammatory cytokines.

The relevance of these findings to OA is unknown because rheumatoid arthritis and models simulating this condition are quite inflammatory relative to OA.

The different types of thermotherapy are presented in *Table 4.3*.

Precautions and contraindications

As with cryotherapy, the greatest concern is with excessive application i.e. in the case of heat therapy, burns. Electric heating pads must be closely monitored! Contraindications include: cardiac insufficiency, malignancy, fever, areas of hypoperfusion, acute inflammation, and hemorrhage. Use caution with superficial heat treatment in areas of edema and open wounds.

THERAPEUTIC EXERCISES

Active and passive exercise programs are beneficial for the OA patient through improvement of muscle strength, joint stability, ROM, and aerobic fitness. Improving these functions is intended to reduce pain and disability. Therapeutic exercise should include stretching and ROM, aerobic conditioning, muscle strength and endurance training, and correction of gait abnormalities. Increasing intensity and duration per session should be implemented in a stepwise fashion until aerobic activity is maintained for 25–30 minutes per treatment session.

Treatment to enhance joint mobility consists of ROM and stretching. Passive ROM is implemented with the patient in lateral recumbency in a quiet and comfortable area. The target joint(s) is slowly and gently flexed and extended until the patient shows initial signs of discomfort, such as tensing the limb, moving, vocalizing, turning the head toward the therapist, or trying to pull away. The therapist should 'challenge' the ROM limits, but not cause undue discomfort. Typically, 15–20 repetitions, performed 2–4 times daily, are adequate.

Stretching is actually an extension of ROM exercises, designed to increase flexibility of tissues. Application of superficial heat or therapeutic ultrasound (US) before stretching may be advantageous, as less damage to the tissues may occur

Table 4.3 Types of thermotherapy

Modality	Comments
Heat	Generally applied for 15–30 min, with equal time off
Hot packs	Heat is absorbed mostly by skin and subcutaneous fat Most packs retain heat for approximately 30 min
Heat wraps	Commercially available for noncanine species May retain low level heat for up to 8 hr
Whirlpool	Patients with chronic conditions may use warmer water (range: 27–35°C) Provides the advantage of hydrostatic pressure
Warm water hosing	More commonly used for equine patients[25]

if the tissues are warmed first. The stretch should be applied at the end of available ROM for at least 15 seconds to encourage elongation of the limiting soft tissue structures to increase available joint motion. Each targeted muscle group should be stretched 3–5 times per session, and 2–4 sessions per day is common.

Active ROM exercises include walking, walking in water, and swimming. More 'demanding' walking activities include walking in snow, sand, tall grass, and crawling through a play tunnel. Climbing stairs and walking over cavaletti rails further develop joint excursions of selected joints and increases strength. As the patient demonstrates continued improvement with therapeutic exercises, strength and endurance are developed. Generally, endurance, cardiovascular fitness, and obesity are addressed through endurance activities. With progression, activities are modified first by increasing the frequency of activity, then by modifying the length of activities, and finally by increasing the speed. A reasonable rule of thumb is to increase the length of activity by 10–15% per week. Further, it is better to provide multiple short duration sessions rather than one extended session when initiating a therapeutic exercise program.

Leash walking

Leash walking is commonly performed incorrectly. Walking an animal slowly encourages the use of all limbs in a sequenced gait pattern (**4.4**). However, the walk must be slow enough to allow weight bearing; if too fast, the animal tends to simply hold the compromised limb up in a flexed, non-weight bearing position. Slow leash walks encourage placement of each limb on the ground, increasing stance time and weight bearing. When appropriate, exercise on a leash can be altered to include fast walking, slow jogging, and running on a long lead. Faster walks further challenge balance, coordination, proprioception, and cardiorespiratory endurance, as well as functional muscle strengthening and endurance (**4.5-4.7**).

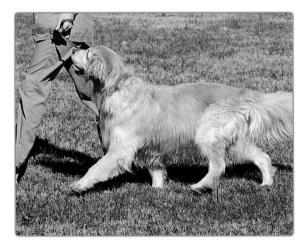

4.4 Slow leash walking encourages limb placement, increased stance time, and weight bearing.

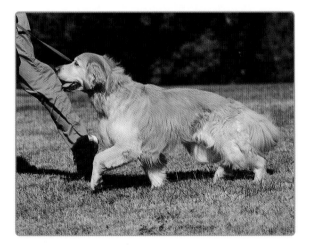

4.5 Faster leash walking promotes muscle strengthening and endurance.

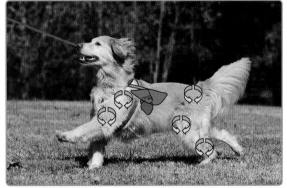

4.6 Fast leash walking promotes cardiorespiratory conditioning and general minor-to-moderate extended range of motion for all joints.

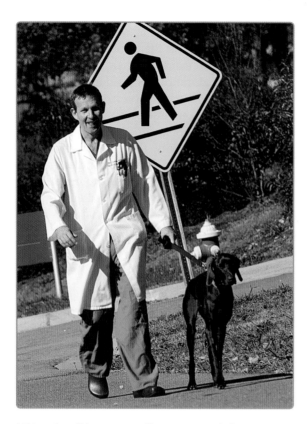

4.7 Leash walking on a gradient promotes balance, proprioception, strengthening, and proper limb placement.

the animal's balance just enough so the animal can recover, being careful not to force the animal to fall.

With a rebound-weight shift, the animal is gently pushed toward the affected side. When the animal shifts its weight to resist the movement, pressure is suddenly released, and gentle pressure is simultaneously applied toward the unaffected side. This results in a sudden unbalancing; the animal initially shifts its weight toward the unaffected side, but to keep from falling, it immediately shifts its weight back toward the affected side. Weight shifts may also be performed during walking. As the animal is walked in a straight line, the handler gently bumps or pushes the animal to one side to challenge the dog to maintain its balance.

When a limb is lifted and held, the animal shifts its body weight in response to this alteration in center of gravity. To maintain the unassisted position, the animal is required to use strength, coordination, and balance. The handler may lift each leg separately to see where the animal is weakest, and focus on that area in subsequent treatment sessions.

A platform on rockers (balance platform or biomechanical ankle platform system [BAPS]) may be used to rock a patient forward and backward, side to side, diagonally and through 360°. With

Walking through a field of tall grass enhances muscle strengthening and endurance, because of the resistance provided by the grass, as well as coordination to navigate varying terrain. Further, dogs have a tendency to flex their joints to a greater extent as they negotiate the grass. Exercising in sand and snow minimizes concussive forces placed on arthritic joints, while allowing strengthening of supporting periarticular muscles (**4.8**).

Weight shifting

Static balance refers to the animal's ability to maintain balance while the body is stationary, such as while standing. Dynamic balance refers to the animal's ability to maintain balance while the body is moving, such as while walking. Exercises performed to challenge the animal's balance include encouraged weight-shifting while standing or walking, manual up-loading of a single limb, balance board, and exercise balls and rolls. The goal is to disturb

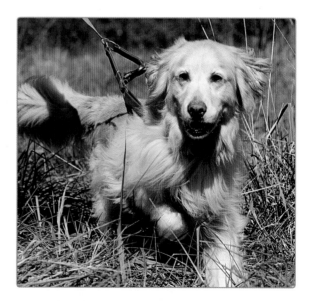

4.8 Leash walking in tall grass, sand, or snow encourages an increased range of joint motion as the animal accommodates to the terrain.

this apparatus, it is important to have one person help support the dog while another person slowly and gently rocks the platform to allow the animal an opportunity to shift its weight and exercise its proprioceptive mechanism (**4.9-4.11**).

Human exercise balls and rolls are easily adapted to animal use (**4.12, 4.13**). The animal's forelimbs are placed on the ball and supported by the handler, requiring the dog to maintain static balance of the

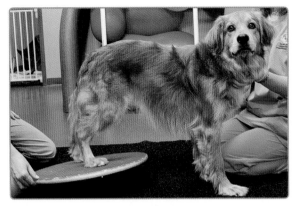

4.11 When using the balance board, one person is attendant to the animal's head, while the other person manipulates the apparatus and assists limb placement.

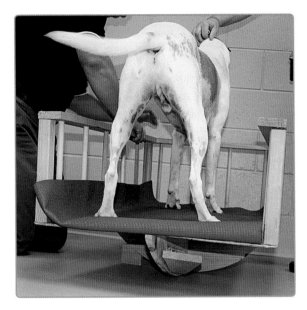

4.9 A rocker platform (teeter board) can be used to rock the patient into a number of positions that help develop its balance and proprioception.

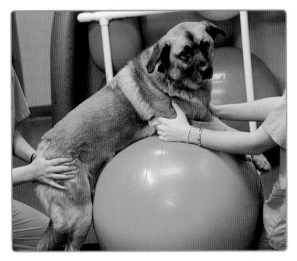

4.12 Physioballs and rolls are excellent aids for balance and proprioception development.

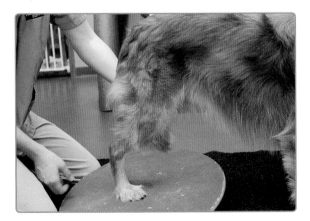

4.10 Balance boards can be used to focus on each individual limb.

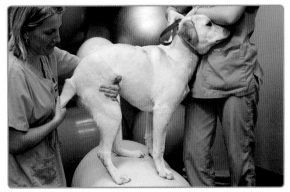

4.13 With appropriate assistance, the physioroll will accommodate standing of small and medium-sized dogs.

caudal trunk and hind limbs. Dynamic balance is challenged as the ball or roll is slowly moved forward, backward, and side to side, challenging the hind legs to maintain balance while movement occurs. In a similar manner, the hind limbs can be placed over the ball to challenge the forelimbs and cranial trunk. Most challenging is to place a dog on an exercise roll with all four limbs in a standing position, while being supported by a handler.

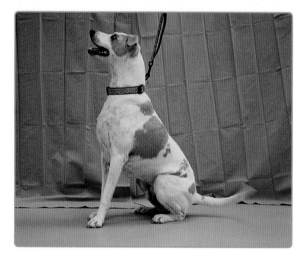

4.14 The sit-to-stand exercise focuses on hind limb muscle group conditioning. Commencing the exercise with the dog positioned in a corner may be helpful if the patient has difficulty controlling its limbs.

Sit-to-stand exercises

Sit-to-stand exercises help strengthen hip and stifle extensor muscles and improve active ROM. The act of sitting, then standing up requires muscle strength of the quadriceps, hamstring, and gastrocnemius muscle groups. This exercise may be particularly beneficial for dogs with OA of the hips. The sit-to-stand exercise allows active contraction of the gluteal muscles, but the hip joint is not generally extended to the point that results in pain. This allows strengthening without creating undue pain (4.14–4.17).

Attention should be paid to sitting and standing straight, with no leaning to one side, and the joints of both hind limbs should be symmetrically flexed so that the dog sits squarely on its haunches. The exercise may be repeated a number of times before the dog is allowed to rest. In some cases it may be easier to back the dog into a corner, with the affected limb next to a wall so that the dog cannot slide the limb out while rising or sitting. Start with 5–10 repetitions once or twice daily, then work up to 15 repetitions 3–4 times daily, using 'empty calorie treats' as required as an incentive. Patients with severe muscle weakness may perform sit-to-stand exercises with sling assistance from a handler or with the pelvis starting from an elevated position,

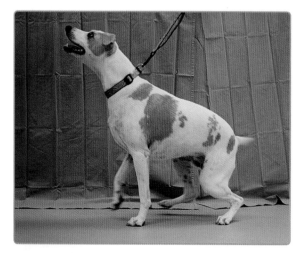

4.15 As the dog begins to rise, contraction is focused on the sartorius, vastus, adductor, and gastrocnemius muscle groups.

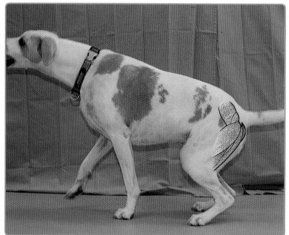

4.16 As the dog continues to rise, the biceps, gluteal, and semitendenosus/membranosus muscle groups are strengthened.

such as on a curb or stool. Sit-to-stands may also be performed in the water to take advantage of the buoyancy of water.

Stairs and steps

Climbing stairs is useful to improve power in the hind limb extensors, ROM, coordination, and balance. Quadriceps and gluteal muscle groups are strengthened as the animal pushes off, extending the hips and tarsus while propelling the body weight up the steps (**4.18**). Begin with 5–7 steps, and gradually increase to 2–4 flights of stairs once or twice daily. Descending stairs improves proprioception and balance, and forelimb strengthening (**4.19**).

Inclines and declines

Weight bearing while climbing promotes extension of the hip joint and flexion of the stifle joint, as well as muscle strengthening (**4.20**). Inclines and declines should be introduced slowly, beginning with gradual slopes, progressing to longer, steeper

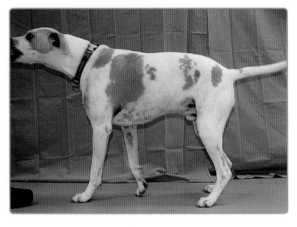

4.17 The dog finishes this exercise in the standing position. 'Empty calorie' treats may be helpful in persuading the dog to perform the sit-to-stand exercise.

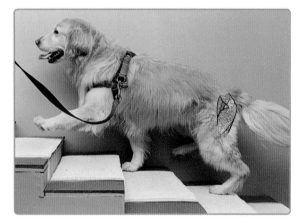

4.18 Ascending steps is a rather complex exercise that conditions the quadricep, hamstring, and gluteal muscle groups.

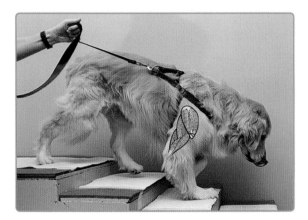

4.19 Descending steps requires balance and proprioception as well as a focus on the forelimb muscle groups. When performing step exercises, ensure a non-skid surface.

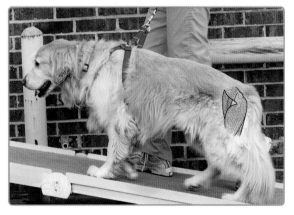

4.20 Inclines focus on extension of both the hip and tarsal joints.

slopes and increasing the duration and speed of the exercise (**4.21**). Walking down slopes is typically more difficult because it requires the animal to reach under its body with the hindlimbs, which requires flexion of the hock and stifle (**4.22**, **4.23**).

Exercising on slopes aids in strengthening of the quadriceps, semitendinosus, semimembranosus, and gluteal muscles with relatively low-impact activity. Muscle strength in the hips and stifles is required for the dog to propel itself up an incline. Further, if the animal's head is held up slightly during the exercise, weight is shifted caudally, requiring the animal to drive up the hill with its hind limbs and challenge these muscles to a greater extent. Corollary effects may be expected in the forelimbs with decline walking.

Dancing and wheelbarrowing

Dancing is a technique to increase weight bearing and force on the hind limbs, while also challenging proprioception, coordination, and balance. When the dog's fore legs are lifted off the ground, this shifts the weight to the hindlimbs and also promotes

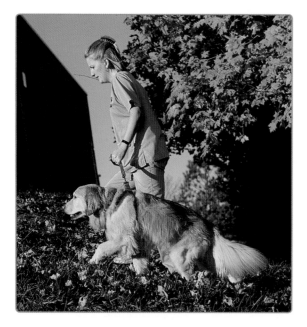

4.21 The 'incline' exercise can be integrated into a leash walk by ascending hills of various gradients.

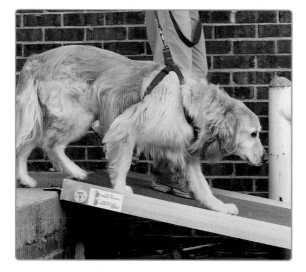

4.22 The 'decline' exercises focus on flexion of the stifle and tarsal joints as the dog reaches under its body with the hindlimbs.

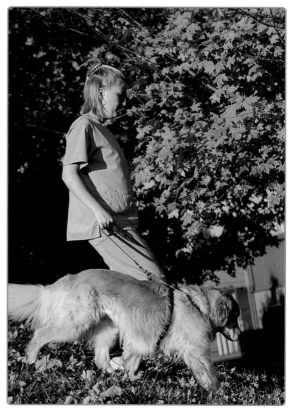

4.23 The 'decline' exercise can be integrated into a leash walk by descending hills of various gradients.

stifle, hock, and hip extension. The higher the dog is elevated off the ground, the more extension is required in the hind limb joints while dancing backwards (4.24–4.26). Dancing in a forward direction results in hip extension similar to that obtained while trotting. Once the dog is capable of using its affected limb consistently at a walk with minimal lameness, it may begin dancing exercises.

How far the dog is elevated off the ground depends on the amount of stress the animal is able to handle comfortably on the hindlimbs. Dogs with normal proprioception will naturally move the hind limbs as the handler moves and the animal 'dances' forward and backward. Dogs may be elevated as high as possible and also dance up and down inclines or hills to place additional stress on the hindlimbs.

Wheelbarrowing is an exercise similar to dancing, except that the forelimbs are targeted. For wheelbarrowing, the handler places the hands under the caudal abdomen and lifts the hind limbs of the dog off the ground, and the dog is moved forward. This exercise encourages increased use of the forelimbs

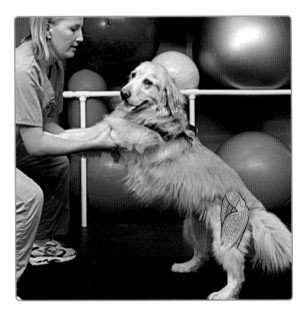

4.24 'Dancing' increases weight-bearing and force on the hind limbs. Dancing at a lower height requires less extension of the hip joint.

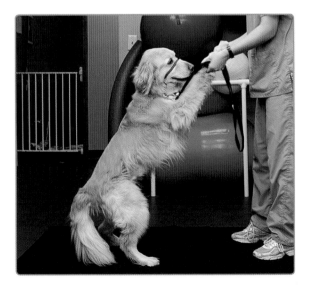

4.25 Dancing at a more medium height can be performed if the dog has a greater range of motion in the hip joint.

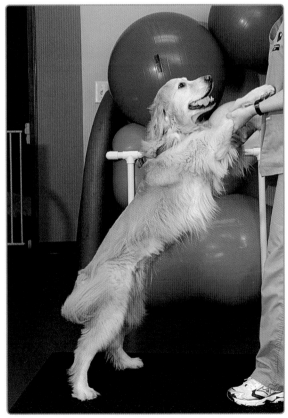

4.26 Dancing in a stretched position requires maximum extension of the hind limb joints.

and challenges proprioception, coordination, and balance (**4.27, 4.28**).

For both dancing and wheelbarrowing, it is advised to muzzle the dog, until the dog demonstrates receptivity to the exercise.

Treadmill activities

Treadmill walking is easily accommodated by dogs that will leash walk. However, they are not used to the ground moving under them, so proprioception, coordination, and balance may be challenged during the first couple of sessions (**4.29**). Treadmills may be useful during initial rehabilitation for conditions in which extension of the hip or stifle is painful, such as hip dysplasia or postoperative recovery from cruciate ligament surgery. Normally, patients are reluctant to perform activities such as climbing stairs, because extension of these joints is painful. Treadmill walking is less painful in some patients because the belt provides assistance with

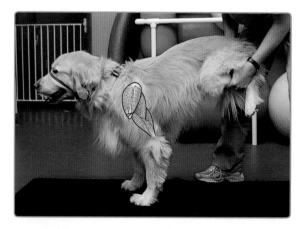

4.27 Wheelbarrow exercises focus on development of the triceps, infra- and supraspinatus muscle groups.

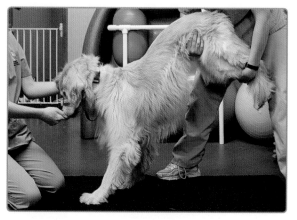

4.28 Administering a 'high' wheelbarrowing exercise challenges the dog's forelimb balance and proprioception.

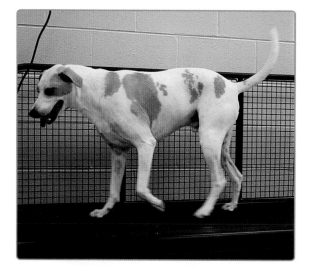

4.29 Treadmill exercise develops proprioception, coordination, and balance. The moving belt assists in hind limb extension.

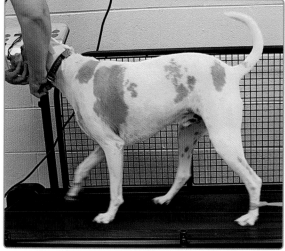

4.30 By attaching an elastic band to the limb, the amount of resistance to forward limb placement can be increased.

hip and stifle extension by helping to pull the hind limb back. There is less need for active contraction of the gluteal and quadriceps muscles for joint extension when walking on a treadmill than when walking on land. For patients with neurologic conditions, the therapist may stand beside the patient and manually advance a foot during the normal gait sequence to encourage gait cadence (**4.30**).

Human-use treadmills may be modified for canine use by adding an overhead bar with a support system to which a canine harness can be attached. The harness helps support the dog in the event it stumbles or falls. Finally, the treadmill may be angled up or down to reduce or increase the forces placed on the forelimbs or hindlimbs.

Cavaletti rails

Cavaletti rails are poles that are spaced apart on the ground at a low height. Cavaletti rails may be used to encourage greater active ROM and lengthening strides in all limbs (**4.31–4.33**). Exercises can be helpful for either orthopedic or neurologic patients in need of improved voluntary motor control and accuracy in placement of their limbs, challenging proprioception, balance, and coordination. After initial Cavaletti rail adaptation, the handler can further challenge the dog by making simple modifications such as adding more poles, increasing the height of all the poles to encourage greater active flexion of joints, and altering the heights of alternating poles to encourage dogs to negotiate

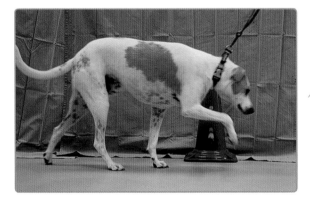

4.31 Cavaletti rails encourage a greater range of motion and lengthening stride.

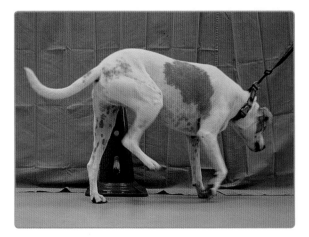

4.33 Cavaletti rails require an increased range of motion in both the forelimbs and hind limbs.

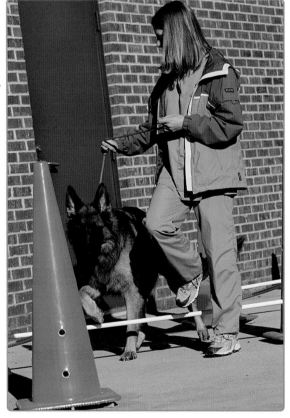

4.32 Exercises using Cavaletti rails encourage development of balance, coordination, and proprioception.

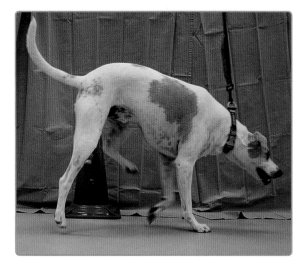

4.34 Cavaletti rails can be raised or lowered to accommodate a desired amount of limb flexion.

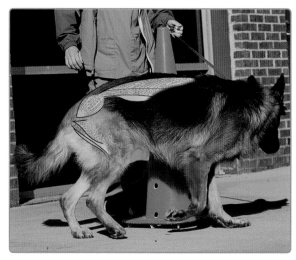

4.35 Pole weaving challenges proprioceptive functioning and strengthens limb abductor and adductor muscles.

different situations (**4.34**). After achieving progress with walking Cavaletti rails, trotting may be introduced.

Pole weaving

Weaving between vertical poles helps to promote side bending of the dog's trunk and also challenges proprioceptive functioning and strengthening of limb abductor and adductor muscles. The handler must lead the animal so that the head, neck, and body actually flex as the poles are negotiated (**4.35, 4.36**). The distance between poles should be adjusted so that sufficient side bending results; in general, the distance between poles should be slightly less than the body length of the dog.

Aquatic exercises

Aquatic therapy takes advantage of several basic principles associated with water: relative density, buoyancy, viscosity, resistance, hydrostatic pressure, and surface tension.

Buoyancy is defined as the upward thrust of water acting on a body that creates an apparent decrease in the weight of a body while immersed. Further, the amount of buoyancy is determined

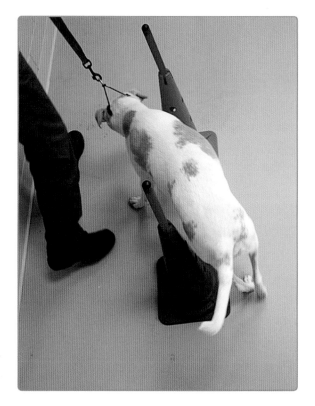

4.36 A dorsal view of pole weaving allows appreciation of the bending of the dog's trunk while navigating the poles.

by how deeply the patient is immersed (**4.37**). Therefore, water allows the patient to exercise in an upright position and may decrease pain by minimizing the amount of weight bearing on joints.

Fluid (hydrostatic) pressure is exerted equally on all surfaces of an immersed body at rest at a given depth in accordance with Pascal's law. This fluid pressure is directly proportional to both the depth and the density of the fluid, i.e. the deeper a body is immersed in water, the greater the pressure exerted. Hydrostatic pressure opposes the tendency of blood

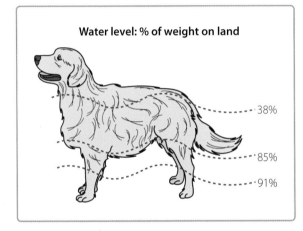

Water level: % of weight on land

38%

85%

91%

4.37 The depth of patient immersion within water determines the amount of 'relative' weight bearing. (Millis DL, Levine D, Taylor RA. *Canine Rehabilitation & Physical Therapy*. 2004. WB Saunders. With permission.)

and edema to pool in the lower portions of the body and can therefore aid in reducing swelling.

The viscosity, or resistance to fluid flow, is significantly greater in water than in air, making it harder to move through water than to move through air. Water can, therefore, provide resistance that may strengthen patient muscles and improve cardiovascular fitness. Surface tension becomes a factor when a limb breaks the surface of the water. Resistance to movement is slightly greater on the surface of water because there is more cohesion on the surface. Therapeutically, if a patient is extremely weak, movements may be performed more easily in the water just beneath the surface rather than at or on the surface.

Studies indicate that pain decreases with aquatic therapy, and active ROM as well as functional ability increase[32]. There are many physiologic effects resulting from exercise in heated water: increased circulation to muscles, increased joint flexibility, and decreased joint pain[32]. If the water temperature is low, peripheral vasoconstriction occurs, blood moves centrally, venous return is enhanced, and stroke volume increases (**4.38–4.42**).

The key to a successful therapeutic exercise program is to have site- and condition-specific exercises whenever possible, to use a variety of exercises and techniques to keep the therapy team and patient from becoming bored, and to allow the animal to progress appropriately so that tissues are

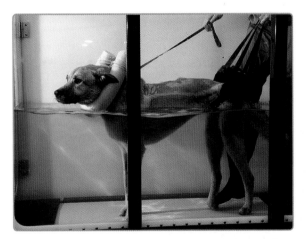

4.38 Buoyancy provided by an underwater treadmill allows excellent facilitation of proprioception training.

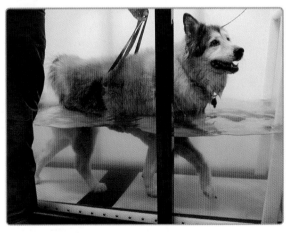

4.39 Underwater treadmill exercising is effective not only for rehabilitation, but also for 'routine fitness'.

adequately challenged for strengthening, but not so rapidly as to result in complications and tissue damage.

OTHER TECHNIQUES

Low-level laser therapy

Low-level laser therapy (LLLT) effects photochemical reactions in the cell (photobiomodulation), exploring the concept that sources of light, such as infrared and ultraviolet light, have therapeutic attributes. Many different types of laser (light amplification by stimulated emission of radiation) are used both industrially and for medical purposes. The lasers used for rehabilitation techniques, LLLT, are also called cold lasers (<100 mW), in contrast to the high power surgical lasers (3000–10,000 mW) designed for thermal destruction of tissues.

Laser light is collimated, coherent and monochromatic. These properties allow low-level laser light to penetrate the skin surface without damage to the skin or heating effect.

Three basic types of lasers are used for LLLT: gaseous HeNe and gallium-arsenide (GaAs) or gallium-aluminum-arsenide (GaAlAs) semiconductor or diode lasers. HeNe lasers emit a visible red light with a wavelength of 632.8 nm, whereas GaAs and GaAlAs emit invisible light near the infrared band with a wavelength of 820–904 nm. Longer wavelengths are more resistant to scattering than are shorter ones; accordingly, GaAs and GaAlAs lasers penetrate more effectively (direct effect up to 2 cm, indirect effect to 5 cm) than HeNe lasers (direct effect up to 0.5 cm, indirect effect up to 1 cm) due to less epidermal and dermal absorption or scattering.

Three variables determine the use of lasers for LLLT: 1) wavelength (typically in the infrared or

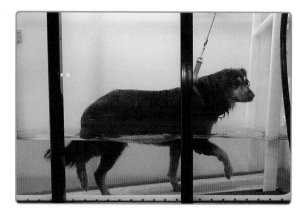

4.40 Underwater treadmills with a variable incline feature take advantage of both the buoyancy and inclined plane features.

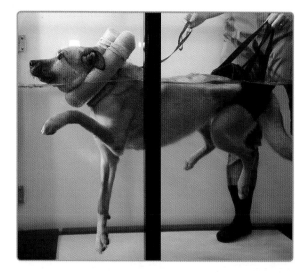

4.41 Increasing the water level to force swimming, encourages a much greater range of motion from all limbs.

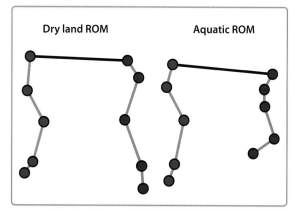

4.42 Kinematic tracings from dogs ambulating both on dry land and immersed in water. An increased range of motion (ROM) is most apparent for the hind limbs from this particular tracing.

near-infrared range of 600–1000 nm); 2) number of watts or milliwatts (typically between 5 and 600 mW); and 3) number of seconds to deliver energy (1–8 J of energy are typically applied to treat various conditions). Given these variables, the time needed to hold the laser probe perpendicular to the treatment area can be calculated[33]. Unfortunately, optimal wavelengths, intensities, and dosages have not been studied sufficiently in animals to determine optimal treatment regimens.

The area of treatment should be clipped free of hair; however, a coupling medium is not necessary, as in US, because the laser beam is not attenuated by air. LLLT should be administered by a trained therapist wearing protective eyewear.

LLLT has been used for the treatment of OA[34–37]; cartilage healing[38]; muscle, ligament, and tendon injuries[39]; wound repair[40,41]; bone healing[42]; and pain relief[43]. Although results from LLLT treatment for pain have been contentious, 635 nm LLLT has been approved by the US Food and Drug Administration for the management of chronic minor pain, as in OA and muscle spasms.

Recent studies in rats have demonstrated the benefits of LLLT in OA and shown that LLLT improves cartilage thickness, decreases cartilage degeneration, and decreases the expression of inflammatory mediators IL-β, capsase-3, matrix metalloproteinase (MMP)-13, and IL-6[44–46]. Multiple studies have also been performed in humans and found that LLLT improves pain scores, ROM, and overall function in humans with chronic knee OA[47–51]. Furthermore, one prospective, double-blind, placebo-controlled study[52] found that elderly patients with knee OA who received an intra-articular injection of hyaluronic acid every 6 months followed by LLLT three times weekly for 6 weeks had a lower need for a total knee replacement when compared to the placebo control group.

Deep heat: shortwave diathermy: ultrasound

Diathermy involves the use of high-frequency oscillating current and US (inaudible sound wave vibrations >20 KHz) to create deep heating. Therapeutic US is a deep-heating modality, effective in heating structures that superficial heat cannot reach. It is useful for improving the extensibility of connective tissue, which facilitates stretching. It is not indicated in acute inflammatory conditions where it may serve to exacerbate the inflammatory response and typically provides only short-term benefit when used in isolation.

US absorption is high in tissues with a high proportion of protein (muscle); however, US waves do not penetrate through air, so it is recommended to clip the hair coat and use appropriate US gel to ensure optimal tissue heating. The duration of US therapy is short, generally 10 minutes, and up to 4 diameters of the sound head may be treated during a session, with 4 minutes of US applied for each sound head diameter. Tissue burns can occur if the intensity is too high or the transducer is allowed to concentrate energy in a small area by stationary positioning. Physes of immature animals should also be avoided. US has been demonstrated to be effective for tendonitis[53,54], joint contracture[55], wound healing[56], and bone healing[57]. Furthermore, recent studies in humans with knee OA have shown that therapeutic US improves overall pain scores, function, and cartilage thickness[58–66].

Extracorporeal shock wave therapy

Extracorporeal shock wave therapy (ESWT) uses very short duration acoustic waves emitted at low frequency (infrasound) and under very high pressure. They have very high energy and are characterized by a peak of very high overpressure (up to 100 times atmospheric pressure), followed by a trough. This occurs very rapidly, within microseconds. Energy is released into tissues when a change in tissue density is encountered, and this energy release is thought to stimulate healing.

Mechanisms explaining the clinical response to ESWT are lacking; however, reported effects include reduced inflammation and swelling, short-term analgesia, improved vascularity and neovascularization, increased bone formation, realignment of tendon fibers, enhanced wound healing and, perhaps, analgesia[67–70]. Research has revealed that ESWT is associated with an increase in bone morphogenetic proteins at fracture sites[69], as well as induction of cytokines and growth factors, such as transforming growth factor β1, substance P, vascular endothelial growth factor, proliferating cell nuclear antigen, and osteocalcin[68].

Francis *et al.* reported the effects of ESWT on hip and elbow OA in dogs[71]. Improvements in weight bearing and comfortable joint ROM were similar to what is typically expected with the use of NSAIDs. Favorable results of ESWT have been reported in dogs by various other authors[72-74]. Shock waves should not be focused on gas-filled cavities or organs due to potential damage to surrounding tissues from energy release, and should not be administered over open growth plates. Heavy sedation or anesthesia is required for most ESWT patients receiving focused shock wave application. Because petechiation/bruising is not an uncommon sequela, concurrent treatment with a COX-1-selective NSAID (aspirin[75], ketoprofin[75], etodolac[75], flunixin meglumine[75], phenylbutazone[75], ± carprofen[76,77] and tepoxaline[78]) is inappropriate. Since ESWT is a localized treatment, a complete understanding of the treatment area anatomy is critical. Only well-trained professionals should administer ESWT; however, the optimal energy level and the number of shocks for various conditions are unknown. Generally, treatments should be repeated no more frequently than every 2 weeks, and most conditions are treated two or three times.

Dogs with immune-mediated joint disease or neurologic deficits should not be treated with ESWT because of unknown effects on these conditions. Neoplastic joint disease, infectious forms of arthritis, and diskospondylitis should not be treated with ESWT because of the risk of spreading the disease.

Electrical stimulation

The goal in using electrical stimulation (ES) for neuromuscular dysfunction is to depolarize a motor nerve (neuromuscular electrical stimulation, NMES) and cause a muscle contraction, whereas the goal for pain management is to depolarize sensory nerves (TENS) to suppress the pain. NMES is used to maintain muscle mass/tone in nonweight-bearing patients. ES electrodes should be applied to clipped skin.

TENS

TENS is a noninvasive therapy mainly used for pain relief for a variety of pain syndromes. Theoretically, high frequency (>50 Hz) and low intensity TENS (HFT) is assumed to work through segmental pain inhibition processes (gate control theory[79]). Low frequency (<10 Hz) and high intensity TENS (LFT) is assumed to be effective by the release of endogenous opioids (suprasegmental effect[80]). Pulse duration and stimulus intensity differ in HFT and LFT and could be decisive factors in efficacy. Both animal and human studies have shown higher analgesic effects by increasing the stimulus intensity or longer pulse duration[81]. Conventional TENS stimulators most commonly used in animals are high frequency (40–150 Hz, 50–100 sec pulse width) and low to moderate intensity because they are more comfortable and create less anxiety in small animal patients.

According to the gate control theory (**4.43**), nociceptive information from small diameter afferents is overridden by stimulation of large diameter fibers, and the pain stimulus is prevented from reaching supraspinal centers. Endogenous opioids released in the central nervous system are also implicated in the analgesic mechanism of TENS. Sluka *et al.* have shown that LFT produces antihyperalgesia by activating central μ-opioid receptors while HFT activates δ-opioid receptors both spinally and supraspinally in the rostral ventromedial medulla[82]. Further, in rats, repeated application of low or high frequency TENS can lead to development of tolerance of spinal μ- and δ-opioid receptors, respectively[83].

In the year 2000, a review of seven trials of TENS and acupuncture-like TENS (AL-TENS) for the treatment of human knee OA concluded that this treatment is effective in managing pain[84]. Levine *et al.* showed, using force-plate analysis, that there was a significant improvement in limb loading of dogs after application of TENS to knees with chronic arthritic impairment[85]. Significant improvement in ground reaction forces was found 30 minutes after treatment, and these differences persisted for 210 minutes after TENS application.

Precautions and contraindications for TENS

High intensity stimulation should be avoided directly over the heart, over areas of impaired sensation, near the abdominal and pelvic regions during pregnancy, over the carotid sinus, or where electrical stimulation might interfere with other electronic sensing devices such as electrocardiography (ECG) monitors.

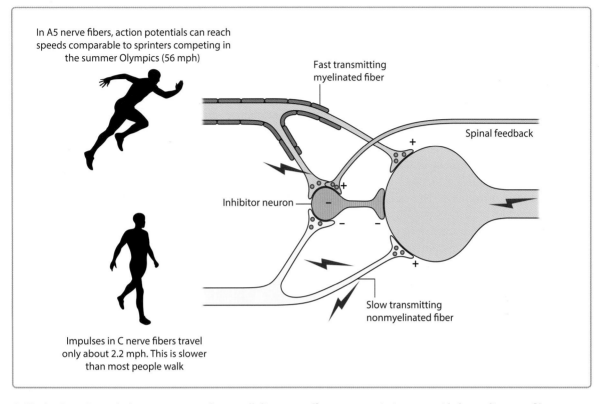

In A5 nerve fibers, action potentials can reach speeds comparable to sprinters competing in the summer Olympics (56 mph)

Fast transmitting myelinated fiber

Spinal feedback

Inhibitor neuron

Slow transmitting nonmyelinated fiber

Impulses in C nerve fibers travel only about 2.2 mph. This is slower than most people walk

4.43 The Gate Control Theory proposes that small diameter afferent transmissions override large diameter fiber transmissions. Signals conducted through the fast transmitting myelinated fiber reach the inhibitor neuron faster than signals from the slow transmitting unmyelinated fiber. The inhibitor neuron then shuts down the transmitter neuron rendering the signal from the slow transmitting unmyelinated fiber ineffective.

TENS applications

Only trained personnel should administer TENS treatment. Patients should be placed in lateral recumbency, muzzled, and may require sedation. Hair is clipped, or the hair is wetted to accommodate fine wire electrodes. Up to four electrodes may be placed over a treatment area. Treatment protocols are empirical; however, application to the desired area(s) for 30 minutes, 3–7 times/week is a common practice. Amperage (intensity) may be slowly increased to the animal's tolerance level, but should be reduced if the patient shows any signs of distress/intolerance.

Acupuncture

Traditional Chinese medicine holds that arthritis is associated with the slowing down in circulation of vital energy (Qi) in meridians surrounding joints.

Further, the water element is involved, perturbing the functions of the kidney, bladder, and the spleen. Kidney function is held to control osteocartilaginous metabolism while spleen function controls joint and periarticular fluids/tissues[86]. Among the various modalities comprising complementary and alternative medicine, acupuncture is perhaps the most deeply scrutinized and investigated[87].

Acupuncture involves the insertion of thin, sterile needles into specific anatomic sites containing a concentration of nerve endings. Expanded forms of acupuncture point stimulation exist, including low-level laser acupuncture therapy, and electroacupuncture, where ES is added to acupuncture treatment. In this way, percutaneous electrical nerve stimulation (PENS) differs from TENS, where electricity must overcome skin resistance, because TENS is delivered by surface electrode pads.

Acupuncture modulates neuron function, inciting a number of responses and reflexes within the peripheral, autonomic, and central nervous systems, with the resultant objective of modulating analgesia[88]. Although acupuncture's mode of action has been explained for centuries in metaphorical and metaphysical terms, its efficacy resides in neurophysiologic alterations, an appreciation that has taken its clinical application from the mystical to the practical. Acupuncture indications and effects, as well as sites for application, are addressed elsewhere[89]. In 2006, Kwon *et al.* critically reviewed 31 possibly relevant studies assessing the effectiveness in humans of acupuncture in peripheral joint OA[90]. Overall, 10 studies demonstrated greater pain reduction in acupuncture groups compared with controls. The authors concluded that considering its favourable safety profile, acupuncture seems an option worthy of consideration for knee OA. In the same year, Habacher *et al.* reported on a systematic review assessing the clinical evidence for acupuncture in veterinary medicine[91]. Fourteen randomized controlled trials and 17 nonrandomized controlled trials were included within their criteria for assessment. Their conclusion was that there is no compelling evidence to recommend or reject acupuncture for any condition in domestic animals. Empirically, results of acupuncture therapy appear to be short-term and, arguably, the greatest value of acupuncture may reside in its complementary effects when administered by well-trained personnel together with other treatment modalities.

Static magnet field

The application of permanent magnets for treating specific human medical problems such as arthritis, chronic pain syndromes, wound healing, insomnia, headache, and others has steadily increased. Magnets marketed directly to consumers are considered safe by the U.S. National Center of Complementary and Alternative Medicine (NCCAM)[92]. Pet owners can purchase magnets that are embedded in wraps, collars, or pet beds.

Results from basic science research demonstrate certain biological effects attributed to static magnet field (SMF), suggesting clinical benefits, namely, increased local blood flow, release of endorphins and anti-inflammatory effects[93–97]. One study on the effect of SMF on relative blood flow to the metacarpus of horses refutes such benefits[98]. Therapeutic magnets range in strength from 2500 to 6000 gauss. (By comparison, the earth's magnetic field is 0.5 gauss, magnetic resonance imaging (MRI) units produce magnetic fields that are 2–4 times that of therapeutic magnets, and common refrigerator magnets are 50–200 gauss.)

In 2007 a critical review of treatment parameters was made for SMF therapy in humans[99]. Among 56 studies reviewed, 61% failed to provide sufficient detail to permit protocol replication by other investigators. This finding illustrates that there are few well-designed, blinded, placebo-controlled studies to evaluate the clinical value of SMF. At present, there is little evidence that this treatment modality has beneficial clinical effects.

MULTIMODAL CASE STUDIES

See *Tables 4.4–4.8* for all data on the following three case studies.

Case 1

Signalment: 'Sara', a 6-year-old, female spayed, 43.6 kg (96 lb), Labrador Retriever, body conditioning score 4/5.

History/presentation: Diagnosed at 9 months of age with bilateral hip dysplasia. At 19 months and weight of 45.45 kg (100 lb), Sara underwent surgical repair of a right cranial cruciate ligament rupture. Two years later, a left cranial cruciate ligament rupture was surgically repaired. Following each cruciate rupture surgery a different NSAID was administered at a 'high-end' dose, but with decreasing efficacy as time progressed. Upon commencing the multimodal protocol, Sara's blood chemistries and urine profiles were unremarkable. Physical examination revealed no abnormalities other than confirmed chronic stifle degenerative joint disease (DJD) and suspected multifocal DJD.

Treatment protocol: Implemented simultaneously:
- Regular, controlled, personalized home exercise program: warm towel application and massage; passive ROM; slow leash walks, with inclines and declines; sit to stand, and balance exercises.

Table 4.4 Range of motion (ROM)

Hindlimb	Normal ROM	Start-Left	Start-Right	11–12 weeks Left	11–12 weeks Right	Change Left	Change Right
Hip Flexion Extension	55° 160–165°	50/55/65 135/151/140	50/44/60 150/148/145	60/60/60 160/160/160	60/46/60 150/151/160	10/5/-5 25/9/20	10/2/NC NC/3/15
Stifle Flexion Extension	45° 160–170°	40/35/55 140/145/150	50/34/65 135/135/135	60/44/40 160/146/165	60/44/45 145/161/160	20/9/-15 20/1/15	10/10/-20 10/26/25
Tarsus Flexion Extension	40° 170°	30/51/* 165/145/*	60/55/* 160/140/*	45/54/* 165/154/*	60/57/* 165/151/*	15/3/* NC/9/*	NC/2/* 5/11/*
Forelimb	**Normal ROM**	**Start-Left**	**Start-Right**	**11–12 weeks Left**	**11–12 weeks Right**	**Change Left**	**Change Right**
Shoulder Flexion Extension	30–60° 160–170°	45/56/* 165/145/*	30/49/* 155/149/*	45/59/* 160/150/*	45/55/* 160/159/*	NC/3/* -5/5/*	15/6/* 5/10/*
Elbow Flexion Extension	20–40° 160–170°	30/35/* 165/160/*	30/40/* 146/160/*	45/40/* 165/167/*	30/44/* 165160/*	15/5/* NC/7/*	NC/4/* 19/NC/*
Carpus Flexion Extension	20–35° 190–200°	30/45/* 195/142/*	30/50/* 195/148/*	35/46/* 190/151/*	35/41/* 190/159/*	5/1/* -5/9/*	5/-9/* -5/11/*

Note: The straight joint position is considered to be 180°.

Data in cells, left to right: Sara/Lois/Koda. *Not noted; NC: no change

Normal Range of Motion Source: Millis DL, Levine D, Taylor RA. *Canine Rehabilitation & Physical Therapy*. Sanders, St. Louis, 2004, p. 441. Range of motion estimates may vary, depending on the source.

Table 4.5 Force plate gait analysis

	Start	Start	At 11–12 weeks	At 11–12 weeks
Foot	Peak vertical force	Vertical impulse	Peak vertical force	Vertical impulse
Right front	25.91/135.4/*	8.018/16.29/*	23.78/133.71/*	8.24/15.39/*
Left front	26.29/132.7/*	8.6616.54/*	24.12/142.06/*	8.15/17.52/*
Right rear	5.99/69.0/38.8	1.73/7.04/5.34	8.66/74.11/43.1	2.92/7.57/6.3
Left rear	13.49/61.5/51.49	4.52/6.74/8.19	9.12/72.96/62.7	3.12/8.93/10.22

Data in cells, left to right: Sara/Lois/Koda

Sara data (units): Peak vertical force (kg/cm^2); vertical implse (kg*sec)

Lois and Koda data (units): Z peak force (100*N/N); Z impulse (area) (100*N-sec/N)

*Not noted

Table 4.6 Overall pain scoring

Start	After 11–12 weeks				
Joint	Start Left	Start Right	After 11–12 weeks left	After 11–12 weeks right	Pain scoring
Hip	2/3+/1	2/3+/1	1/1/0	1/1/0	0 = No pain on palpation
Stifle	2/0/2	2/0/2	1/1/0	1/1/0	1 = Mild pain; palpation completed
Tarsus	0/0/*	2/0/*	0/0/*	0/0/*	2 = Moderate pain; palpation completed with obvious discomfort noted
Shoulder	1/0/*	0/0/*	0/0/*	0/0/*	3 = Severe pain; palpation not completed
Elbow	0/0/*	0/1/*	0/0/*	0/0/*	4 = Pain too severe; restraint/ sedation needed to paplate
Carpus	0/0/*	0/0/*	0/0/*	0/0/*	
Data in cells, left to right: Sara/Lois/Koda					
*Not noted					

Table 4.7 Overall subjective lameness

	Start	After 11–12 weeks	
Sara	2	1	
Lois	4	1	**Scale** 1= None/mild; 5= Severe
Koda	4	1	

Table 4.8 Gait assessment (stance and movement)

		Start	After 11–12 weeks	Scoring
Sara				0 = Normal stance
	at stance	2	1	1 = Slightly abnormal stance (partial weight bearing)
	at walk	3	0–1	2 = Moderately abnormal stance (toe-touch weight bearing)
	at trot	2	1	3 = Severely abnormal stance (holds limb off floor)
Lois				4 = Unable to stand
	at stance	2+	0	
	at walk	2+	0	0 = No lameness; full weight bearing on all strides
	at trot	2+	1	1 = Mild subtle lameness with partial weight bearing
Koda				2 = Obvious lameness with partial weight bearing
	at stance	2	1	3 = Obvious lameness with intermittent weight bearing
	at walk	2	1	4 = Full non-weight-bearing lame
	at trot	3	1	

- High eicosapentaenoic acid (EPA) diet only: 2 cups (454 g; 16 oz) (maximum) of dry Hills' J/D diet per day.
- Eight dose protocol (label) of polysulfated glycosaminoglycan (Adequan® Canine).
- Daily NSAID administration: 100 mg deracoxib.

Results:
- ROM was improved in 79% of the joints, as assessed by goniometer.
- Force plate gait analysis did not show improved changes as demonstrable as the subjective clinical improvements.
- Sara's owner was extremely pleased with her dog's improvement resultant from the multimodal protocol, with comments such as, "When Sara goes outside now, she comes in running like a streak of lightning through the house," and "Sara had another great day!"
- Striving to achieve the 'minimal effective dose' of the NSAID; the NSAID dose was decreased by 50% after 6 weeks on the multimodal protocol, and another 50% (to 25 mg SID) after 11 weeks.
- The patient's blood/chemistry profiles and urine assessments were unchanged over the course of the multimodal treatment protocol.

Veterinarian and Affiliation: Larry Baker DVM, FAVD, DAVDC: Northgate Pet Clinic, Decatur IL, USA.

Case 2
Signalment: 'Lois', a 13.7-year-old, female spayed, 21.3 kg (47 lb), Labrador Retriever, body condition score 2.8/5.

History/presentation: At an early age, Lois developed ovariohysterectomy incontinence, which was 'somewhat' successfully being managed with phenylpropanolamine hydrochloride at 50 mg BID. At approximately 3 years of age, she was diagnosed with lumbosacral disease, and had received a few, intermittent steroid injections over the lumbosacral area, which provided relief for acute symptoms. Lois' owner attributed her weight loss to a reluctance to walk to the food bowl. Physical examination revealed a stiff gait, poor muscle mass, a wide-based hind limb stance, preference to walk on surfaces with 'good footing', and a painful response to manipulation of the hips and lumbosacral spine. Blood work was normal. Radiographs revealed mild hip dysplasia, a narrowing of the lumbosacral intervertebral disc space, and lumbosacral spondylosis.

Treatment protocol: Treatment goal was to manage pain, increase muscle strength, and modify progression of lumbar facet DJD by:
- Daily NSAID administration: 31 mg/day (1.46 mg/kg) for the first 4 days only, then 25 mg (1.17 mg/kg) once daily thereafter.
- Exclusive diet of Hills' dry and canned J/D diet.
- Polysulfated glycosaminoglycan (Adequan® Canine) at 4.4 mg/kg Q4–5 days for eight injections, then Q21 days for two injections, and thereafter Q4–5 weeks PRN.
- Regular leash walks with modest inclines and declines; brisk walking/jogging in grass, and sit-to-stand exercises. Massage of the lower back and hips was encouraged, together with warm and cold therapy before and after exercise, respectively.
- Acupuncture was suggested, but declined, and inclusion of tramadol PRN was anticipated.

Results:
- Over the course of 12 weeks Lois gained approximately 0.8 kg (2 lb).
- Over the 12-week treatment protocol, increased ROM was noted in all joints of the hind limb.
- Force plate gait analysis showed an improvement of weight bearing in all limbs excepting the right fore. Asymmetry between the hind limbs was reduced from 8% (clinically relevant) to 1% (nonclinical).
- Lois' owner was not aggressive with therapeutic exercises, not striving for an active pet, but rather simply to increase Lois' comfort. However, a huge improvement in leash walking was noted. Lois' average walk of only 60 m (a few hundred feet), 3–4 times per day, increased to approximately 1.6 km (1 mile) per day. Further, Lois became more willing and able to go up and down stairs, doing so with clearly greater ease and confidence. Overall improvement was noted immediately upon commencement of treatment and further improvement was seen with time.

- The patient's blood/chemistry profiles and urine assessments were unchanged over the course of the multimodal treatment protocol.

Veterinarian and Affiliation: Alan S. Gassel DVM: Concord Veterinary Hospital, Farragut TN, USA.

Case 3

Signalment: 'Koda', a 9-year-old, female spayed, 30 kg (60 lb), Labrador Retriever, body conditioning score 3/5.

History/presentation: Following surgical repair (extracapsular) of bilateral cranial cruciate ligament tears at ages 1 and 3 years, and normal aging as an active dog, Koda was losing her ability to fully participate in a rural, active lifestyle that included running, hunting, swimming, and rigorous activity with other dogs. Following exercise, she would become stiff and suffer exacerbated lameness for at least 24 hr. Prior to implementing this multimodal protocol, Koda was treated conservatively with weight control and various 'traditional' NSAIDs. Koda's blood chemistries and urine profiles were within normal limits. Physical examination was unremarkable, excepting severe, chronic DJD of both stifles and mild DJD of both coxofemoral joints, each diagnosis confirmed by radiographs. She was taking glucosamine sulfate (750 mg PO SID).

Treatment protocol:
- High EPA diet of Hills J/D diet.
- Eight dose protocol (label) of polysulfated glycosaminoglycan (Adequan® Canine).
- Daily NSAID administration: 50 mg deracoxib (decreased to 37 mg, i.e. 1.7 mg/kg to 1.2 mg/kg).
- Nutraceutical: glucosamine sulfate (750 mg SID).

Results:
- Over the course of 11 weeks, Koda gained 1.5 kg (3.3 lb).
- Only the hip and stifle were assessed for ROM. Extension of both the hips and stifle were improved by approximately 10–13%.
- Based upon force plate gait analysis, there appeared to be marked improvement in the left hind limb. Improvement in the right hind limb was also noted, but was less dramatic. Koda's

owner believed that she (Koda) once again had the opportunity to enjoy 'a summer on the lake' which she had been unable to do for the past couple of years.
- The NSAID dose was reduced from 1.7 mg/kg to 1.2 mg/kg SID.
- The patient's blood/chemistry profiles and urine assessments were unchanged over the course of the multimodal treatment protocol.
- Following this multimodal treatment protocol, the owner has stated, "Koda has been observed running her 'sprints' around the yard, has been on several 3.2 km (2 mile) runs without tiring or becoming lame, has been eager to play fetch, and has actually fought our daughter's 3-year old Labrador for the right to retrieve sticks in the water. It has been wonderful to see her playing tug-of-war with the younger dog! The most impressive change, however, has been the absolute lack of stiffness/lameness the day following vigorous activity at the lake. We attribute this improvement, at least in part, to the NSAID therapy; as when this medication has occasionally been forgotten, stiffness has been particularly noticeable."

Veterinarian and Affiliation: Dr. Heather Hadley: Michigan State University, East Lansing MI, USA.

REFERENCES

1 Zhang W, Moskowitz RW, Nuki G, *et al.* OARSI recommendations for the management of hip and knee osteoarthritis, part 1: critical appraisal of existing treatment guidelines and systematic review of current research evidence. *Osteoarthr Cartilage* 2007;**15**:981–1000.

2 McMaster W. A literary review on ice therapy in injuries. *Am J Sports Med* 1977;**5**:124–6.

3 Olson J, Stravino V. A review of cryotherapy. *Phys Ther* 1972;**62**:840–53.

4 Hayes K. Cryotherapy. In: *Physical agents*, edn 4. Appleton & Lange, Norwalk, 1993, pp. 9–15.

5 Millis DL. Physical therapy and rehabilitation in dogs. In: Gaynor JS, Muir WM (eds). *Handbook of Veterinary Pain Management*, edn 2. Mosby Elsevier, St. Louis, 2002, p. 508.

6 Drez D, Faust DC, Evans JP. Cryotherapy and nerve palsy. *Am J Sports Med* 1981;**9**:256–7.

7 Bassett FH III, Kirkpatrick JS, Englehardt DL, *et al*. Cryotherapy-induced nerve injury. *Am J Sports Med* 1992;**20**:516–18.

8 Nadler SF, Weingand KW, Stitik TP, *et al*. Pain relief runs hot and cold. *Biomechanics* 2001;**8**:1.

9 Myrer JW, Measom G, Fellingham GW. Temperature change in the human leg during and after two methods of cryotherapy. *J Athletic Training* 1998;**33**:25–9.

10 Zemke JE, Andersen JC, Guion WK, *et al*. Intramuscular temperature responses in the human leg to two forms of cryotherapy: ice massage and ice bag. *J Orthop Sports Phys Ther* 1998;**27**:301–7.

11 Ho SS, Coel MN, Kajawa R, *et al*. The effects of ice on blood flow and bone metabolism in knees. *Am J Sports Med* 1994;**22**:537–40.

12 Brosseau L, Yonge KA, Robinson V, *et al*. Thermotherapy for treatment of osteoarthritis. *Cochrane Database Syst Rev* 2003, issue 4, Art. No: CD004522. DOI: 10.1002/14651858.CD004522.

13 Howatson G, Van Someren KA. Ice massage, effects on exercise-induced muscle damage. *J Sports Med Phys Fitness* 2003;**43**:500–5.

14 Drygas KA, McClure S, Goring RL, *et al*. Prospective evaluation of cold compression therapy on postoperative pain, swelling, range of motion, and lameness following tibial plateau leveling osteotomy in dogs. 2009; in press. *J Am Vet Med Assoc* 2011;**15**(10):1284–91.

15 Moeller JL, Monroe J, McKeag DB. Cryotherapy-induced common peroneal nerve palsy. *Clin J Sport Med* 1997;**7**:212–16

16 Petrov R, MacDonald MH, Tesch AM, *et al*. Influence of topically applied cold treatment on core temperature and cell viability in equine superficial digital flexor tendons. *Am J Vet Res* 2003;**64**:835–44.

17 Hayes K. Cryotherapy. In: *Physical Agents*, edn 4. Appleton & Lange, Norwalk, 1993, pp. 49–59.

18 Hing WA, White SG, Bouaaphone A, *et al*. Contrast therapy: a systematic review. *Phys Ther Sport* 2008;**9**:148–61.

19 Myrer JW, Draper DO, Durrant E. Whirlpool contrast therapy. *J Athletic Training* 1994;**29**:318–22.

20 Myrer JW, Measom G, Durrant E, *et al*. Cold- and hot-pack contrast therapy: subcutaneous and intramuscular temperature change. *J Athletic Training* 1997;**32**:238–41.

21 Bassett FH, Kirkpatrick JS, Engelhardt DL, *et al*. Cryotherapy-induced nerve injury. *Am J Sport Med* 1992;**20**:516–18.

22 Saxena A. Achilles peritendinosis: an unusual case due to frostbite in an elite athlete. *J Foot Ankle Surg* 1994;**33**:87–90.

23 Sallis R, Chassay CM. Recognizing and treating common cold-induced injury in outdoor sports. *Med Sci Sports Exerc* 1999;**31**:1367–73.

24 Vannatta ML, Millis DL, Adair S, *et al*. Effects of cryotherapy on temperature change in caudal thigh muscles of dogs [abstract]. In: Marcellin-Little DJ (ed). *Proceedings of the Third International Symposium on Rehabilitation and Physical Therapy in Veterinary Medicine*. Department of Continuing Education, NC State College of Veterinary Medicine, Raleigh, 2004, p. 205.

25 Kaneps AJ. Superficial cold and heat. In: Levine D, Millis DL (eds). *Proceedings of the Second International Symposium on Rehabilitation and Physical Therapy in Veterinary Medicine*. University of Tennessee, University Outreach and Continuing Education, Knoxville, 2002, pp. 41–7.

26 Cameron MH. Thermal agents: cold and heat. In: *Physical Agents in Rehabilitation: From Research to Practice*, edn 3. Elsevier Health Sciences, Philadelphia, 2008, pp. 1312–77.

27 Reid RW, Foley JM, Prior BM, *et al*. Mild topical heat increases popliteal flood flow as measured by MRI. *Med Sci Sports Exerc* 1999;**31**:S208.

28 Erasala GN, Rubin JM, Tuthill TA, *et al*. The effect of topical heat treatment on trapezius muscle blood flow using power Doppler ultrasound. *Phys Ther* 2001;**81**:A5.

29 Davis KD, Kwan CL, Crawley AP, *et al*. Functional MRI study of thalamic and cortical activations evoked by cutaneous heat, cold, and tactile stimuli. *J Neurophysiol* 1998;**80**:1533–46.

30 Nadler SF, Steiner DJ, Erasala GN, *et al*. Continuous low level heat wrap therapy provides more efficacy than ibuprofen and acetaminophen for acute low back pain. *Spine* 2002;**27**:1012–14.

31 Markovic M, Stuhlmeier KM. Short-term hyperthermia prevents activation of

proinflammatory genes in fibroblast-like synoviocytes by blocking the activation of the transcription factor NF-kappaB. *J Mol Med* 2006;**84**:821–32.

32 Templeton MS, Booth DL, O'Kelly WD. Effects of aquatic therapy on joint flexibility and functional ability in subjects with rheumatic disease. *J Orthop Sports Phys Ther* 1996;**23**:376–81.

33 Millis DL, Francis D, Adamson C. Emerging modalities in veterinary rehabilitation. *Vet Clin North Am (SAP)* 2005;**35**(6):1335–55.

34 Stelian J, Gil I, Habot B, *et al.* Laser therapy is effective for degenerative osteoarthritis: improvement of pain and disability in elderly patients with degenerative osteoarthritis of the knee treated with narrow-band light therapy. *J Am Geriatr Soc* 1991;**40**:23–6.

35 Djavid GE, Mortazavi SMJ, Basirnia A, *et al.* Low-level laser therapy in musculoskeletal pain syndromes: pain relief and disability reduction. *Lasers Surg Med* 2003;**152**:43.

36 Gur A, Cosut A, Sarac AJ, *et al.* Efficacy of different therapy regimes of low-power laser in painful osteoarthritis of the knee: a double-blind and randomized-controlled trial. *Lasers Surg Med* 2003;**33**:330–8.

37 Tascioglu F, Armagan O, Tabak Y, *et al.* Low power laser treatment in patients with knee osteoarthritis. *Swiss Med Wkly* 2004;**134**:254–8.

38 Guzz GA, Tigani D, Torricelli P, *et al.* Low-power diode laser stimulation of surgical osteochondral defects: results after 24 weeks. *Artif Cells Blood Substit Immobil Biotechnol* 2001;**29**:235–44.

39 Fung DT, Ng GY, Leung MC, *et al.* Therapeutic low energy laser improves the mechanical strength of repairing medial collateral ligament. *Lasers Surg Med* 2002;**31**:91–6.

40 Mester E, Spiry T, Szende B, *et al.* Effect of laser rays on wound healing. *Am J Surg* 1971;**122**:532–8.

41 Enwemeka CS, Parker JC, Dowdy DS, *et al.* The efficacy of low-power lasers in tissue repair and pain control: a meta-analysis study. *Photomed Laser Surg* 2004;**22**:323–9.

42 Barber A, Luger JE, Karpf A, *et al.* Advances in laser therapy for bone repair. *Laser Ther* 2001;**29**:80–5.

43 Bjordal JM, Couppé C, Chow R, *et al.* A systematic review of low-level laser therapy with location-specific doses for pain from chronic joint disorders. *Aus J Physiother* 2003;**49**:107–16.

44 Alves ACA, Albertini R, dos Santos SA, *et al.* Effect of low-level laser therapy on metalloproteinase MMP-2 and MMP-9 production and percentage of collagen types I and III in a papain cartilage injury model. *Lasers Med Sci* 2014;**29**:911–19.

45 Assis L, Milares LP, Almeida T, *et al.* Aerobic exercise training and low-level laser therapy modulate inflammatory response and degenerative process in an experimental model of knee osteoarthritis in rats. *Osteoarthr Cartilage* 2016;**24**(1):169–77.

46 Dos Santos SA, Alves ACA, Leal-Junior ECP, *et al.* Comparative analysis of two low-level laser doses on the expression of inflammatory mediators and on neutrophils and macrophages in acute joint inflammation. *Lasers Med Sci* 2014;**29**:1051–58.

47 Alfredo PP, Bjordal JM, Dreyer SH, *et al.* Efficacy of low level laser therapy associated with exercises in knee osteoarthritis: a randomized double-blind study. *Clinical Rehabilitation* 2011;**26**(6):523–33.

48 Alghadir A, Omar MTA, Al-Askar AB, *et al.* Effect of low-level laser therapy in patients with chronic knee osteoarthritis: a single-blinded randomized clinical study. *Lasers Med Sci* 2014;**29**:749–55.

49 Hegedus B, Viharos L, Gervain M, *et al.* The effect of low-level laser in knee osteoarthritis: a double-blind, randomized, placebo-controlled trial. *Photomed Laser Surg* 2009;**27**(4):577–84.

50 Nakamura T, Ebihara S, Ohkuni I, *et al.* Low level laser therapy for chronic knee joint pain patients. *Laser Therapy* 2014;**23**(4):273–77.

51 Soleimanpour H, Gahramani K, Taheri R, *et al.* The effect of low-level laser therapy on knee osteoarthritis: prospective, descriptive study. *Lasers Med Sci* 2014;**29**:1695–1700.

52 Ip D, Fu NY. Can combined use of low-level lasers and hyaluronic acid injections prolong the longevity of degenerative knee joints. *Clin Interven Aging* 2015;**10**:1225–58.

53 Enwemeka CS, Rodriguez O, Mendosa S. The biomechanical effects of low-intensity ultrasound on healing tendons. *Ultrasound Med Biol* 1990;**16**:801–7.

54 Saini NS, Roy KS, Bansal PS, *et al.* A preliminary study on the effect of ultrasound therapy on the

healing of surgically severed Achilles tendons in five dogs. *J Vet Med Physiol Pathol Clin Med* 2002;**49**:321–8.

55 Loonam JE, Millis DL. The effect of therapeutic ultrasound on tendon healing and extensibility. In: *Proceedings of the 30th Annual Conference of the Veterinary Orthopedic Society*. Veterinary Orthopedic Society, Newmarket, 2002, p. 69.

56 Dyson M, Pond JB, Joseph J, *et al.* The stimulation of tissue regeneration by means of ultrasound. *Clin Sci* 1968;**35**:273–85.

57 Warden SJ. A new direction for ultrasound therapy in sports medicine. *Sports Med* 2003;**33**:95–107.

58 Cakir S, Hepguler S, Ozturk C, *et al.* Efficacy of therapeutic ultrasound for the management of knee osteoarthritis: a randomized, controlled, and double-blind study. *Am J Phys Med Rehabil* 2014;**93**:405–12.

59 Langer MD, Levine V, Taggart R, *et al.* Pilot clinical studies of long duration, low intensity therapeutic ultrasound for osteoarthritis. *Proc IEEE Annu Northeast Bioeng Conf.* 2014; doi:10.1109/NEBEC.2014.6972850

60 Loyola-Sanchez A, Richardson J, Beattie K, *et al.* Effect of low-intensity pulsed ultrasound on the cartilage repair in people with mild to moderate knee osteoarthritis: a double-blinded, randomized, placebo-controlled pilot study. *Arch Phys Med Rehabil* 2012;**93**:35–42.

61 MacIntyre NJ, Busse JW, Bhandari M. Physical therapists in primary care are interested in high quality evidence regarding efficacy of therapeutic ultrasound for knee osteoarthritis: a provincial survey. *Sci World J* 2013;1–7. http://dx.doi.org/10.1155/2013/348014

62 Mascarin NC, Vancini RL, Andrade MS, *et al.* Effects of kinesiotherapy, ultrasound and electrotherapy in management of bilateral knee osteoarthritis: prospective clinical trial. *BMC Musculoskel Dis* 2012;**13**:182.

63 Ozgonenel L, Aytekin E, Durmusoglu G. A double-blind trial of clinical effects of therapeutic ultrasound in knee osteoarthritis. *Ultrasound Med Biol* 2009;**35**:44–9.

64 Srbely JZ. Ultrasound in the management of osteoarthritis: part I: a review of the current literature. *J Can Chiropr Assoc* 2008;**52**(1):30–7.

65 Yang PF, Li D, Zhang SM, *et al.* Efficacy of ultrasound in the treatment of osteoarthritis of the knee. *Orthopaedic Surgery* 2011;**3**(3):181–7.

66 Zeng C, Li H, Yang T, *et al.* Effectiveness of continuous and pulsed ultrasound for the management of knee osteoarthritis: a systemic review and network meta-analysis. *Osteoarthr Cartilage* 2014;**22**:1090–99.

67 Thiel M. Application of shock waves in medicine. *Clin Orthop* 2001;**387**:18–21.

68 Ogden JA, Alvarez RG, Levitt R, *et al.* Shock wave therapy (orthotripsy) in musculoskeletal disorders. *Clin Orthop* 2001;**387**:22–40.

69 Wand CJ, Wand FS, Yang KD, *et al.* Shock wave therapy induces neovascularization at the tendon-bone junction: a study in rabbits. *J Orthop Res* 2003;**21**:984–9.

70 Wang FS, Yang KD, Kuo YR, *et al.* Temporal and spatial expression of bone morphogenetic proteins in extracorporeal shock wave-promoted healing of segmental defect. *Bone* 2003;**32**:387–96.

71 Francis DA, Millis DL, Evans M, *et al.* Clinical evaluation of extracorporeal shockwave therapy for the management of canine osteoarthritis of the elbow and hip joints. In: *Proceedings of the 31st Meeting Veterinary Orthopedic Society*. Veterinary Orthopedic Society, Okemos, 2004.

72 Becker W, Kowaleski MP, McCarthy RJ, *et al.* Extracorporeal shockwave therapy for shoulder lameness in dogs. *J Am Anim Hosp Assoc* 2015;**51**:15–19

73 Dahlberg J, G Fitch G, Evans RB, *et al.* The evaluation of extracorporeal shockwave therapy in naturally occurring osteoarthritis of the stifle joint in dogs. *Vet Comp Orthop Traumatol* 2005;**18**:147–52.

74 Mueller M, Bockstahler B, Skalicky M, *et al.* Effects of radial shockwave therapy on the limb function of dogs with hip osteoarthritis. *Vet Rec* 2007;**160**:762–65.

75 Ricketts AP, Lundy KM, Seibel SB, **et al.** Evaluation of selective inhibition of canine cyclooxygenase 1 and 2 by carprofen and other nonsteroidal anti-inflammatory drugs. *AJVR* 1998;**59**:1441–6.

76 Brainard BM, Meredith CP, Callan MB, *et al.* Changes in platelet function, hemostasis, and prostaglandin expression after treatment with nonsteroidal anti-inflammatory drugs with

various cyclooxygenase selectivities in dogs. *AJVR* 2007;**68**:251–7.

77 Wooten JG, Blikslager AT, Ryan KA, *et al.* Cyclooxygenase expression and prostanoid production in pyloric and duodenal mucosae in dogs after administration of nonsteroidal anti-inflammatory drugs. *AJVR* 2008;**69**:457–64.

78 Zubrin (tepoxalin). Technical monograph; Schering–Plough Animal Health 2003.

79 Melzack R, Wall PD. Pain mechanisms: a new theory. *Science* 1965;**150**:971–9.

80 Walsh DM. *TENS: Clinical Application and Related Theory.* Churchill Livingstone, New York, 1997.

81 Garrison DW, Foreman RD. Effects of transcutaneous electrical nerve stimulation (TENS) on spontaneous and noxiously evoked dorsal horn cell activity in cats with transected spinal cords. *Neurosci Lett* 1996;**216**:125–8.

82 Sluka KA, Deacon M, Stibal A, *et al.* Spinal blockade of opioid receptors prevents the analgesia produced by TENS in arthritic rats. *J Pharmacol Exp Ther* 1999;**289**:840–6.

83 Chandran P, Sluka KA. Development of opioid tolerance with repeated transcutaneous electrical nerve stimulation administration. *Pain* 2003;**102**:195–201.

84 Osiri M, Welch V, Brosseau L, *et al.* Transcutaneous electrical nerve stimulation for knee osteoarthritis. *Cochrane Database of Systematic Reviews 2000*, Issue 4. Art. No: CD002823. DOI: 10.1001/14651858. CD002823.

85 Levine D, Johnston KD, Price MN, *et al.* The effect of TENS on osteoarthritic pain in the stifle of dogs. In: *Proceedings of the 2nd International Symposium on Rehabilitation and Physical Therapy in Veterinary Medicine.* University of Tennessee, Knoxville, 2002, p. 199.

86 Molinier F. *Traité d'Acupuncture Vétérinaire.* Editions Phu Xuan, Paris, 2003.

87 Pascoe PJ. Alternative methods for the control of pain. *JAMVA* 2002;**221**:222–9.

88 Staud R, Price DD. Mechanisms of acupuncture analgesia for clinical and experimental pain. *Expert Rev Neurother* 2006;**6**:661–7.

89 Robinson N. Complementary and alternative medicine for pain management in veterinary patients. In: Gaynor JS, Muir WW (eds). *Handbook of Veterinary Pain Management,* edn 2. Mosby Elsevier, St. Louis, 2002, pp. 301–15.

90 Kwon YD, Pittler MH, Ernst E. Acupuncture for peripheral joint osteoarthritis: a systematic review and meta-analysis. *Rheumatology* 2006;**45**:1331–7.

91 Habacher G, Pittler MH, Ernst E. Effectiveness of acupuncture in veterinary medicine: systematic review. *J Vet Intern Med* 2006;**20**:480–8.

92 https://nccih.nih.gov/health/magnet/magnetsforpain.htm

93 Markov MS, Pilla AA. Weak static magnetic field modulation of myosin phosphorylation in a cell-free preparation: calcium dependence. *Bioelectrochem Bioenerg* 1997;**43**:233–8.

94 McKay JC, Prato FS, Thomas AW. A literature review: the effects of magnetic field exposure on blood flow and blood vessels in the microvasculature. *Bioelectromagnetics* 2007;**28**:81–98.

95 Taniguchi N, Kanai S, Kawamoto M, *et al.* Study on application of static magnetic field for adjuvant arthritis rats. *Evid Based Compl Alt Med* 2004;**1**:187–91.

96 Xu S, Tomita N, Ikeuchi K, *et al.* Recovery of small-sized blood vessels in ischemic bone under static magnetic field. *Evid Based Compl Alt Med* 2007;**4**:59–63.

97 Morris CE, Skalak TC. Chronic static magnetic field exposure alters microvessel enlargement resulting from surgical intervention. *J Appl Physiol* 2007;**101**:629–36.

98 Steyn PD, Ramey DW, Kirschvink J, *et al.* Effect of a static magnetic field on blood flow to the metacarpus of horses. *JAVMA* 2000; **217**:874–8.

99 Colbert AP, Wahbeh H, Harling N, *et al.* Static magnetic field therapy: a critical review of treatment parameters. *eCAM* 2007; DOI:10.1093/ecam/nem131.

Chapter 5

Regenerative Medicine for Multimodal Management of Canine Osteoarthritis

Brittany Jean Carr, DVM, CCRT

Sherman O. Canapp, DVM, MS, CCRT Diplomate ACVS, Diplomate ACVSMR

REGENERATIVE MEDICINE FOR OSTEOARTHRITIS

While osteoarthritis (OA) is a common cause of pain and lameness in dogs, no definitive treatment has been identified. In many dogs, conservative treatments including non-steroidal anti-inflammatory medications (NSAIDs), joint supplements, weight management, and rehabilitation therapy fail to provide a long-term response. For these patients, regenerative medicine is another option in the multimodal approach to managing OA.

The use of regenerative medicine has been used to stimulate healing in areas that have not responded to more traditional approaches. Every tissue has the capacity to either heal or scar after injury. While some tissues are able to heal back to their original strength and resilience, other tissues such as cartilage heal poorly. The goal of regenerative medicine is to help the body regenerate injured tissue back to its original condition. Regenerative medicine has been used to decrease pain and inflammation and to promote cartilage function and healing in patients with OA.

PLATELET-RICH PLASMA

Platelet-rich plasma (PRP) is an autogenous fluid concentrate composed primarily of platelets and growth factors. Recent studies have shown PRP to mediate healing by supplying growth factors, cytokines, chemokines, and other bioactive compounds[1-7]. Initially PRP's first clinical applications were limited to dentistry and maxillofacial surgery to improve bone healing. However, PRP currently has much broader clinical applications, extending to orthopedic surgery and sports medicine. PRP is currently used in both people and animals to help with healing in numerous tissues. Recent studies have shown PRP to be efficacious in managing many different orthopedic conditions, including OA and soft tissue injuries[3,4,7-31]. Thus, numerous commercial PRP point-of-care technologies have become available.

Platelets play roles in both hemostasis and wound healing. Platelets contain granules that release growth factors to stimulate other cells of the body to migrate to the area of trauma, thus facilitating tissue healing. It is the growth factors contained within the platelets that are of significance for tissue healing (*Table 5.1*). These growth factors include platelet-derived growth factor (PDGF), transforming growth factor (TGF)-β1, TGF-β2, vascular endothelial growth factor (VEGF), basic fibroblastic growth factor (bFGF), and epidermal growth factor (EGF)[1-4,6]. Many of these growth factors have been shown to act either individually or synergistically to enhance cellular migration and proliferation, angiogenesis and matrix deposition to promote tendon and wound healing, aid in cartilage health, and counteract the cartilage breakdown that is associated with OA[2-8,10-13,19- 22,26,29,31]. Platelets have also been shown to recruit, stimulate, and provide a scaffold for stem cells[27,31-39]. Thus, PRP has been used as a regenerative medicine therapy to aid in tissue healing.

Multiple formulations of PRP have been developed and studied. Previous studies in humans have reported that the ideal PRP product should have any-

Table 5.1 The effect of growth factors on cartilage/chondrocytes, synovium, and mesenchymal stem cells.

Growth factor	Chondrocytes/ cartilage	Synovium	Mesenchymal stem cell	References
TGF-β1	Stimulates synthesis of ECM. Decreases catabolic activity. of IL-1 and MMPs.	Causes synovial proliferation and fibrosis. Induces chemotaxis of inflammatory leukocytes to synovium. Induction of osteophyte formation.	Increases proliferation and ECM production. Downregulates collagen type 1 gene expression.	127–133
BMP-2	Stimulates synthesis of ECM. Partial reversal of dedifferentiated phenotype in OA. Increased ECM turnover (increased aggrecan degradation).	Presumed role in maturation of osteophytes. Multiple injections lead to synovial fibrosis. Stimulates synovial thickening in experimental OA.	Increases proliferation and ECM production. Downregulates collagen type 1 gene expression.	129, 131–134
BMP-7	Stimulates ECM synthesis. Decreases cartilage degradation through decreasing activity/ expression of numerous ILs and MMPs.	Decreases expression of MMPs and aggrecanase. Does not appear to cause osteophyte formation or synovial fibrosis.	Inhibits cell proliferation. Inconsistent ability to induce chondrogenesis alone. Potentiates chondrogenic differentiation with TGF-βs resulting in increased ECM synthesis and decreasing collagen type 1 compared with TGF-β alone.	135–139
IGF-I	Stimulates ECM synthesis. Decreases matrix catabolism except in aged and OA cartilage.	Protective effect on synovium resulting in decreased thickening and decreased evidence of chronic inflammation.	Stimulates cell proliferation. Increases expression of ECM. Additive effect when combined with TGF-β.	140–143
FGF-2	Decreases aggrecanase activity. Antagonizes PG synthesis. Upregulates MMPs.	Induces synovial proliferation. Inflammatory and induces osteophyte formation when used alone.	Increases PG synthesis. Increases cell proliferation.	144–147
FGF-18	Increases chondrocyte proliferation and stimulates ECM *in vitro* and in injured joints but not in normal joints.	Induces synovial thickening. Enlargement of chondrophytes in experimental OA.		147–149
PDGF	No adverse effect in normal joints.	No adverse effect in normal joints.	Induces proliferation.	150, 151

TGF-β1 = transforming growth factor-β1; BMP = bone morphogenetic protein; IGF-I = insulin growth factor I; FGF = fibroblast growth factor; PDGF= platelet-derived growth factor; ECM = extracellular matrix; IL = interleukin; MMP = matrix metalloproteinase; OA = osteoarthritis.

Ref: Fortier LA, Barker JU, Strauss EJ, *et al.* The role of growth factors in cartilage repair. *Clin Orthop Relat Res* 2011;**469**:P2706–2715.

where from a 4- to 7-fold increase in platelets[2-4,6]. However, platelet concentration is not the only important component of a PRP product. Inclusion or exclusion of mononuclear cells, neutrophils, and red blood cells (RBC) not only define an autologous platelet product, but also have been reported to affect the clinical efficacy of the product and play major roles affecting the inflammatory responses after PRP injection[2,5,10,19-22,40-44]. In general, it is believed that RBC and neutrophils should be reduced as they have an inflammatory effect, while the effect of mononuclear cells remains largely unknown[36,40,41,45,47,48].

Reducing RBC concentration is thought to be important when developing the ideal PRP product[40]. A recent study revealed an increased RBC concentration in PRP increases the concentrations of unwanted inflammatory mediators, specifically interleukin (IL)-1 and TGF-α. This study also showed that synoviocytes treated with RBC concentrate demonstrated significantly more synoviocyte death when compared with leukocyte-rich PRP (LR-PRP), leukocyte-poor PRP (LP-PRP), and phosphate-buffered saline (PBS.)[40].

The effect of leukocyte concentration in PRP products has also been investigated. Both LR-PRP and LP-PRP have been studied and compared. Recent studies have shown LR-PRP is associated with increased proinflammatory mediators, including IL-1β, IL-6, IL-8, interferon (IFN)-γ, and TNF-α[1,2,5,10,40,41]. Increased leukocytes in PRP are also associated with more marix metalloproteinase (MMP-3 and MMP-13) gene expression and less cartilage oligomeric matrix protein and decorin gene expression[10,36,45]. These potentially deleterious effects are largely attributed to the presence of neutrophils. Additionally, an increased concentration of neutrophils in PRP is also positively correlated with an increased MMP-9 concentration which degrades collagen and other extracellular matrix molecules[20,36,41,45]. One recent study has shown LR-PRP causes significantly more synoviocyte death when compared with LP-PRP and PBS[40]. Thus, LP-PRP has been thought to be more beneficial than LR-PRP in maintaining tendon homeostasis and counteract inflammation associated with OA[10,19,20,40,45,46].

While an increased neutrophil concentration in PRP is known to have negative effects, the effect of monocytes and lymphocytes remains largely unknown. Recent studies suggest that monocytes are associated with an increase in cellular metabolism and collagen production in fibroblasts and a decrease in release of anti-angiogenic cytokines IFN-γ and IL-12[47,48]. Platelets have also been shown to activate peripheral blood mononuclear cells (lymphocytes, monocytes, and macrophages) to help stimulate collagen production, which is believed to be mediated by an increase in IL-6 expression[47,48]. However, the role of monocytes and lymphocytes in PRP therapy remains unclear and further investigation is warranted.

PRP therapy is often performed as a series of 1 to 3 injections with 2 weeks between each injection. If PRP is being used to manage moderate to severe OA, in the authors' experience about 50% of dogs require more than one injection for significant improvement. PRP therapy is a minimally invasive procedure that typically can be performed on an outpatient basis. Approximately 30 to 60 mL of blood is obtained, processed, and prepared for injection (**5.1, 5.2**).

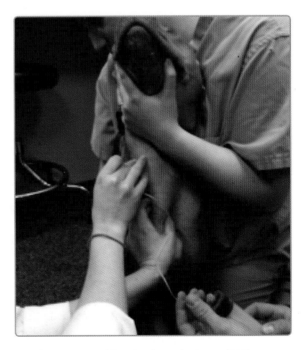

5.1 Blood collected for platelet-rich plasma (PRP) processing using an 18-gauge butterfly needle and syringe. Most systems require anywhere from 10 to 60 mL of blood for PRP processing.

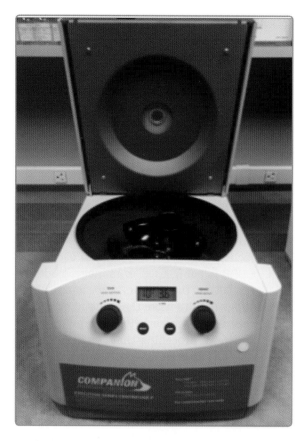

5.2 Both centrifugation and filtration systems are available for platelet-rich plasma (PRP) processing. This is a centrifugation PRP system used for PRP processing that produces a leukocyte- and erythrocyte-poor PRP sample.

Once the PRP is processed, the area that is to be treated is clipped and aseptically prepared. Sedation or general anesthesia may or may not be required, depending on the location of the injection. For OA, PRP joint injections are usually performed without sedation; however, some joints such as the hip require sedation and may also require advanced imaging (fluoroscopy) for guidance.

The most common side effect is discomfort associated with the injection, which typically resolves within 12 to 24 hours of the injection. Mild discomfort occurs in the first 24 to 72 hours following the injection and can be managed with pain medication if needed. NSAIDs and steroids are avoided 2 weeks prior to and post PRP therapy. Finally, a dedicated conditioning program is often recommended in conjunction with PRP therapy to achieve and maintain the fullest musculoskeletal potential and performance level.

Case 1

Signalment: Sasha is a 2-year-old female Rottweiler who was diagnosed with a traumatic left fragmented medial coronoid process that was arthroscopically removed 3 months prior to presentation. She presented for an intermittent left forelimb lameness noted after long walks and at the trot.

Initial Assessment:
Lameness Grade (VI point scale):
  Grade II/VI left thoracic limb lameness present at the trot
Range of Motion:
  Left elbow flexion: 35°
  Left elbow extension: 145°
  Right elbow flexion: 35°
  Right elbow extension: 145°
Gait Analysis:
  Left forelimb TPI%: 26%
  Right forelimb TPI%: 31.2%

Treatment:
Bilateral elbow intra-articular injections of PRP

Results (90 days following treatment):
Lameness Grade (VI point scale):
  No observable lameness present
Range of Motion:
  Left elbow flexion: 35°
  Left elbow extension: 145°
  Right elbow flexion: 35°
  Right elbow extension: 145°
Gait Analysis:
  Left forelimb TPI%: 29.8%
  Right forelimb TPI%: 30%

Sasha's owner reported that she was able to go for long walks without any observable lameness. She was very pleased with her progress and Sasha was released to return to full activity at that time.

STEM CELL THERAPY

Stem cells are the body's progenitor cells from which all other cells are derived. Recent studies have shown that stems cells can regenerate and heal injured tissue, decrease inflammation, stimulate new blood supply to support healing, activate resident stem cells, create a scaffold for healing tissue, protect cells from death, and break down scar tissue[49–55]. The mechanisms by which these cells initiate healing within the body are complex. Mesenchymal stem cells (MSCs) decrease pro inflammatory and increase anti-inflammatory mediators. MSCs are activated to become immunosuppressive by soluble factors and in turn secrete factors that inhibit T-lymphocyte activation and proliferation[49–55]. MSCs secrete bioactive levels of cytokines and growth factors that support angiogenesis, tissue remodeling, differentiation, and anti-apoptotic events[49–55]. The cytokines and growth factors secreted by the MSCs can also assist in neovascularization[49–55]. MSCs demonstrate a diverse plasticity and are able to help regenerate injured tissues.

Recent studies have demonstrated the efficacy of stem cell therapy for the treatment of canine OA. One recent study in dogs with elbow OA caused by spontaneous fragmented coronoid process demonstrated that dogs who underwent arthroscopic fragment removal and a proximal ulnar ostectomy and received either stromal vascular fraction (SVF) or allogeneic stem cells had a more favorable outcome than dogs who were treated with surgery alone[56]. Another recent study demonstrated that dogs with hip OA who received a single intra-articular injection of adipose derived cultured progenitor cells (ADPC) had a better outcome than control patients and patients who received plasma rich in growth factors (PRGF)[57]. Similarly, other recent studies also demonstrated superiority of osteoarthritic dogs treated with ADPC over control patients and those treated with PRGF on controlled, blinded force platform analysis[58,59].

Stem cells can be obtained from numerous sources from a patient's own body (autologous adult-derived mesenchymal cells). The most common places to harvest adult-derived mesenchymal cells are either from the patient's bone marrow or adipose tissue. Both bone marrow-derived and adipose-derived stem cells have the ability to differentiate into cartilage, bone, tendons, and ligaments. To date, there is no evidence to support superiority of one over the other in terms of viability or efficacy of the derived stem cells.

Once the sample is obtained, it is then processed and prepared for injection. Both bone-marrow derived stem cells and adipose-derived stem cells can be processed either on-site or shipped for processing, culturing, and banking for future use[60]. As with other forms of regenerative medicine, stem cell therapy is a minimally invasive procedure that typically can be performed on an outpatient basis with or without the use of sedation, depending on the location of the injection. Also, since recent studies have shown that PRP recruits and stimulates stem cells, PRP is often combined with stem cells prior to injection to both activate and act as a scaffold for the stem cells (5.3)[60–67].

ADIPOSE-DERIVED STEM CELL THERAPY

Adipose tissue is often a common source of stem cells in dogs as it is easily obtainable with little donor site morbidity and patient discomfort. Sites for adipose collection include: the falciform ligament and subcutaneous fat deposits of the thoracic wall, caudal to the scapula, and inguinal region. A recent study evaluated patient factors influencing the concentration of mesenchymal cells in SVF[68]. In this study, age significantly affected the viable cells per gram (VCPG) with younger dogs having a significantly higher VCPG than older dogs. Also, adipose tissue collected at the falciform location had

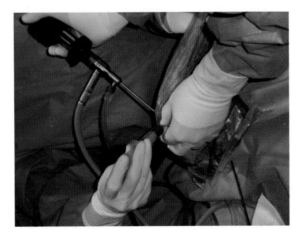

5.3 An intra-articular stifle injection of bone marrow aspirate concentrate and platelet-rich plasma in a patient with moderate osteoarthritis.

significantly fewer VCPG than tissue collected at the thoracic wall and inguinal locations. Neutered dogs also had significantly fewer VCPG in tissue collected at the falciform location than at the thoracic wall and inguinal locations when compared to intact dogs. Thus, specific patient factors should be taken into consideration in order to obtain the maximal yield of VCPG from an adipose collection procedure. In the authors' experience, the falciform ligament is preferred for obtaining an adequate fat sample as there is less morbidity and the procedure is more cosmetic.

Adipose-derived cultured progenitor cells

ADPC are cells that are harvested and then isolated, cultured, and expanded prior to injection. Typically 10–20 g of adipose tissue is collected and shipped to a laboratory for isolation, culturing, and expansion (**5.4, 5.5a,b**).

A number of validated techniques to produce viable progenitor cells exist for ADPC. This is done in a controlled environment with compliance to safety and processing standards. ADPC culturing and expansion yields a homogenous cell population of anywhere from 5 to 10 million total viable

mesenchymal cells[68]. Residual cells are often banked for future use using a validated method, as a recent study has shown that long-term cryopreservation does not effect adipogenic, osteogenic, or myogenic

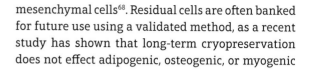

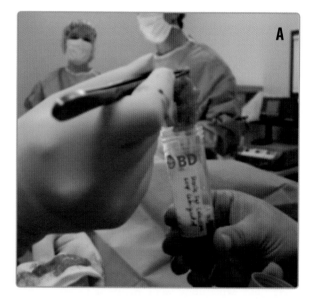

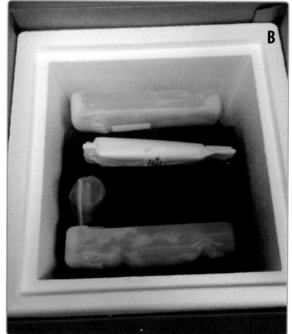

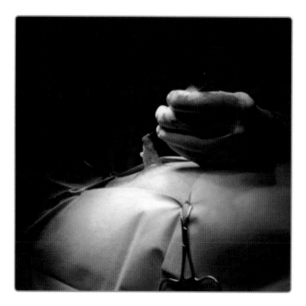

5.4 Collection of adipose tissue from the falciform ligament for stromal vascular fraction processing.

5.5a,b Adipose being prepared for shipment to the laboratory for processing.

differentiative potential[60]. The disadvantages of ADPC include the need to ship the cells to and from the laboratory and the time required for isolation, culturing, and expansion (typically 14–21 days). Also, since the cells are manipulated, they may be considered a "drug" by the Food and Drug Administration (FDA) in the future, which would mandate inclusion under FDA regulations.

Stromal vascular fraction

The SVF contains mesenchymal cells that have been isolated from a fat sample that is mechanically and/or enzymatically digested and processed. While less literature is available regarding the efficacy of SVF when compared to ADPC, SVF is commonly used clinically as it can be collected, processed in-house, and administered all on the same day. Typically 20–50 g of adipose tissue is collected and processed in-house without extensive manipulation of the cells, allowing for same-day treatment. To minimize the risk of cell contamination, it is essential that the cells are processed in a clean environment with a high level of safety and control standards. The average SVF system yields a heterogenous population of cells with a total viable cell count anywhere from 8 to 41 million, depending on the system used[68,69]. Residual cells may or may not be able to be banked, depending upon the system used and the capabilities of, and the resources available to, the clinic at which they are processed.

BONE MARROW-DERIVED STEM CELL THERAPY

Bone marrow is commonly used as a source for stem cells, as it is relatively easy to collect. Bone marrow is typically collected from the proximal femur, ilium, or humerus under heavy sedation or anesthesia (**5.6**).

In the authors' experience, the proximal femur is preferred, as large samples of bone marrow can be easily obtained with relatively low morbidity.

Cultured bone marrow-derived stem cells

Cultured bone marrow derived stem cells (BMSC) contain mesenchymal cells that are isolated from a sample of bone marrow, cultured, and expanded in a laboratory setting. Typically 5–10 mL of bone marrow is collected and shipped to the laboratory for isolation, culturing, and expansion. A number of validated techniques to produce viable progenitor cells exist for culture expanded BMSC. Similar to ADPC, this is done in a controlled environment with safety and processing standards and takes 14 to 21 days. Residual cells are often banked for future use using a validated method, as a recent study has shown that long-term cryopreservation does not effect adipogenic, osteogenic, or myogenic differentiative potential[60]. The same disadvantages for ADPC exist for culture expanded BMSC.

Bone marrow aspirate concentrate

Bone marrow is also a common source in dogs, as it is easily obtained with little donor site morbidity and patient discomfort. Sites for bone marrow collection include the proximal femur, the proximal humerus, and the ilium. Typically 30–60 mL of bone marrow is required for processing. BMAC contains mesenchymal cells that are mechanically isolated

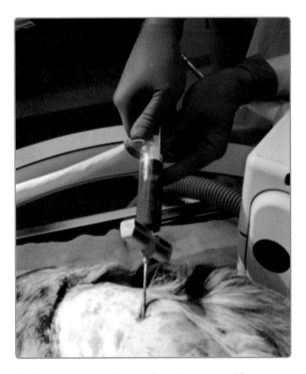

5.6 Bone marrow collection from the proximal femur with fluoroscopic guidance for bone-marrow aspirate concentrate processing.

and concentrated from a sample of the patient's bone marrow (**5.7**).

While the sample can be processed either in-house or mailed to a commercial laboratory, there are multiple in-house BMAC systems available for veterinary use, which makes same-day treatment possible. However, there is still limited validation data available for these systems. Published data report that the average BMAC system can produce anywhere from 1,000 to 10,000 MSC/mL[69–71].

RECOMMENDATIONS FOLLOWING STEM CELL THERAPY

Following stem cell therapy, recommendations for post-procedural care and rehabilitation therapy are made. NSAIDs and steroids are avoided for at least 8 weeks following stem cell therapy, as they are thought to inhibit stem cell differentiation, proliferation, and migration[72–74]. Cold compressing the affected area is also discouraged as stem cell differentiation is slowed *in vitro* under cold conditions[75,76]. Rehabilitation therapy with manual therapy, class IIIb low-level laser therapy (LLLT), and therapeutic exercise is recommended to be performed weekly for the first 12 weeks following stem cell therapy.

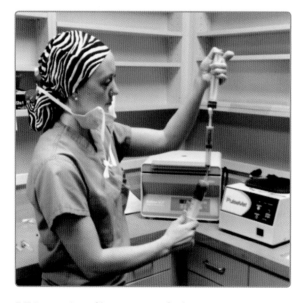

5.7 Processing of bone marrow for bone marrow aspirate concentrate using an in-house system that mechanically separates and concentrates mesenchymal cells.

Class IIIb LLLT is recommended as it has been shown to stimulate stem cell differentiation, proliferation, and viability *in vitro*[77–82]. The effects of class IV LLLT on stem cells remain unknown; thus, class IV LLLT is discouraged for the first 8 weeks following stem cell therapy. Similarly, all other rehabilitation therapy modalities (therapeutic ultrasound, electrotherapy, etc.) are discouraged for the first 8 weeks following stem cell therapy, as their effect on stem cell viability and differentiation has not been fully studied.

Case 2
Signalment: Brogan is a 12-year-old, castrated male Sheltie, who presented for a left forelimb lameness secondary to moderate-to-severe left elbow OA. Brogan underwent left elbow arthroscopy. A fragmented medial coronoid process was noted and grade IV–V cartilage erosion of the medial compartment was noted at the time of arthroscopy. Fragment excision and abrasion arthroplasty was performed. In spite of participation in a dedicated rehabilitation therapy program and implementing various other intra-articular therapies, Brogan's left forelimb lameness and left elbow discomfort persisted.

Initial Assessment:
Lameness Grade (VI point scale):
    Grade III/VI left thoracic limb lameness present
Range of Motion:
    Left elbow flexion: 50°
    Left elbow extension: 145°
    Right elbow flexion: 50°
    Right elbow extension: 145°
Gait Analysis:
    Left forelimb TPI%: 27%
    Right forelimb TPI%: 32%

Treatment: Left elbow intra-articular injection of SVF and PRP.

Results (90 days following treatment):
Lameness Grade (VI point scale):
    Grade I/VI left thoracic limb lameness present
Range of Motion:
    Left elbow flexion: 40°
    Left elbow extension: 145°
    Right elbow flexion: 40°
    Right elbow extension: 145°

Gait Analysis:
  Left forelimb TPI%: 29%
  Right forelimb TPI%: 30%

At the 90-day re-evaluation, Brogan's owner reported that he is more comfortable at home and able to play and participate in activities that he previously could not. Overall, she was very pleased with his progress.

OTHER INTRA-ARTICULAR THERAPIES

Interleukin-1 receptor antagonist protein

IL-1 receptor antagonist protein (IRAP) is an endogenous protein that inhibits IL-1 activity by binding to the IL-1 receptor, which prevents IL-1 ligand/receptor interactions and downstreaming signaling events that play an integral role in the progression of inflammation associated with OA[83]. IRAP therapy has been used in humans as well as rabbits, dogs, and horses with OA[84-94]. Thus, numerous systems have become available for veterinary use to produce IRAP, which can be administered intra-articularly to reduce IL-1 signaling that potentiates inflammatory pathways associated with OA. These systems are designed to increase the expression of leukocyte-derived IL-1RA by incubating clotted whole blood within a chamber containing borosilicate beads. The serum is then collected, filtered, and administered intra-articularly. Recent studies have evaluated the use of these systems and validated large increases in IL-1RA and other anti-inflammatory proteins[95,96]. Other studies have validated their efficacy and showed improved comfort and function in patients treated with IRAP[91-93]. One recent study reported dogs with unilateral elbow or stifle OA that received one single intra-articular injection of IRAP had significantly improved lameness scores, pain scores, and peak vertical force at 12 weeks following injection when compared to pretreatment values[94].

Hyaluronic acid

Viscosupplementation with hyaluronic acid (HA) for the treatment of OA is based on improving the rheologic properties within the joint as previous studies have shown that there is a decrease in molecular weight and concentration of HA in arthritic joints[97-103]. HA has been shown to slow the progression of OA, decrease inflammation within the joint, and have chondroprotective effects. Specifically, it increases the joint fluid viscosity, increases cartilage (glycosaminoglycan: GAG) formation, and decreases degradative enzymes and cytokines[104-109]. Intra-articular HA has been widely used in the treatment of OA in animals and humans. Several clinical studies in humans have demonstrated relief of joint pain associated with OA following intra-articular injections of HA[110-113]. Information regarding the effects of intra-articular HA on naturally occurring OA in dogs is not available; however, several experimental studies using intra-articular HA in dogs have been reported. Results from these studies have demonstrated decreases in pain, lameness, osteophytosis, synovial hyperemia and hypertrophy, GAG and cartilage degradation[114-118]. The mechanism by which HA produces beneficial effects remains controversial.

Studies evaluating the effects of intra-articular HA have used doses ranging from 10 to 20 mg and treatment periods ranging from 3 to 16 weekly injections. One recent study that evaluated the efficacy of 2 mL of 20 mg/mL intra-articular low-molecular weight HA for knee OA showed no difference in outcome between patients who received HA weekly for 3 weeks versus patients who received HA weekly for 6 weeks[119]. Thus, the current recommendation for intra-articular HA therapy for OA is to administer HA once weekly for 3 weeks (**5.8**).

Complications from these injections may include temporary increased pain and lameness and septic

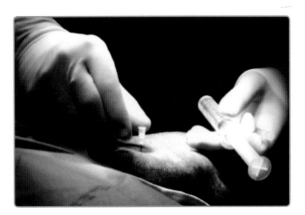

5.8 An intra-articular elbow injection of hyaluronic acid in a patient with elbow arthritis.

arthritis. Recent studies have suggested that high molecular weight, cross-linked HA is not superior to low molecular weight and had double the frequency of post-injection joint flares[120,121]. Reportedly, over 70% of dogs respond well to HA and improvement can be noted for over 6 months following administration[122].

Case 3

Signalment: Duke is a 1.5-year-old, castrated male Labrador Retriever. Duke was diagnosed with bilateral elbow dysplasia and suspected fragmented medial coronoid processes. Bilateral elbow arthroscopy was performed and revealed bilateral fragmented medial coronoid processes with a modified Outerbridge score of a grade 1 in the right elbow and grade 2 in the left elbow. Duke presented 6 months following bilateral elbow arthroscopy for a persistent intermittent left forelimb lameness.

Initial Assessment:
Lameness Grade (VI point scale):
  Grade III/VI left thoracic limb lameness present
Range of Motion:
  Left elbow flexion: 52°
  Left elbow extension: 140°
  Right elbow flexion: 40°
  Right elbow extension: 140°
Gait Analysis:
  Left forelimb TPI%: 24%
  Right forelimb TPI%: 32%

Treatment: Bilateral elbow intra-articular injection of 20 mg of hyaluronic acid once weekly for 3 weeks.

Results (90 days following treatment):
Lameness Grade (VI point scale):
  No observable lameness present
Range of Motion:
  Left elbow flexion: 30°
  Left elbow extension: 140°
  Right elbow flexion: 30°
  Right elbow extension: 140°
Gait Analysis:
  Left forelimb TPI%: 29.2%
  Right forelimb TPI%: 29.2%

Duke's owner was thrilled with the results and reported a great improvement in daily function and overall comfort. Duke was able to go for long walks, hikes, and play in the yard without showing any signs of lameness or discomfort.

Corticosteroids

In humans, intra-articular corticosteroids are recommended in several guidelines for the treatment of patients with OA. Corticosteroids prevent the formation of both prostaglandins and leukotrienes by causing the release of lipocortin, which by inhibition of phospholipase A2, reduces arachidonic acid release. The two most commonly used corticosteroids used as an intra-articular therapy to manage OA are methylprednisolone acetate (Depo-Medrol®) and triamcinolone acetonide (Vetalog®).

Methylprednisolone acetate (Depo-Medrol®)

One study evaluated the use of 20 mg of intra-articular methylprednisolone acetate immediately post transection of the cranial cruciate ligament (CCL), wherein 4-weeks post transection of the CCL showed a chondroprotective effect. The dogs treated with methylprednisolone acetate had a significantly reduced incidence and size of osteophytes, reduced histologic grading of cartilage lesions, and suppression of stromelysin synthesis[123].

Methylprednisolone acetate is available for veterinary use in both 20 mg/mL and 40 mg/mL sterile aqueous suspensions (**5.9**).

The recommended intra-articular dose for dogs is 20 mg for a large synovial space, such as the stifle. Smaller spaces will require a correspondingly smaller dose.

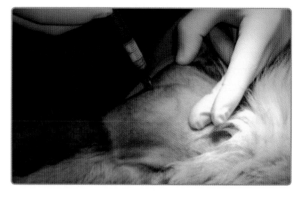

5.9 An intra-articular injection of methylprednisolone acetate in a patient with elbow osteoarthritis.

Triamcinolone acetonide (Vetalog®)

One study evaluated the use of 5 mg of intra-articular triamcinolone immediately post transection of the CCL and at 4- and 8-weeks post transection of the CCL. Dogs who received intra-articular triamcinolone had significantly reduced numbers and size of the osteophytes, reduced histologic severity of cartilage, and reduced expression and synthesis of proteolytic enzymes, such as stromelysin and IL-1[123]. A recent study also compared the effects of triamcinolone and methylprednisolone on cartilage and synovium, suggesting that triamcinolone could have fewer deleterious effects on cartilage and synovium viability compared to methylprednisolone[124].

Triamcinolone acetonide is available for veterinary use in both 2 mg/mL and 6 mg/mL solutions. The recommended intra-articular dose is 1–3 mg.

Clinical use of intra-articular corticosteroids

Corticosteroids are believed to be safe and effective for long-term management of OA. One recent study showed that corticosteroids were safe for repeated use every 3 months for up to 2 years with no joint space-narrowing detected[125]. Side effects of intra-articular administration include transient pain elicited immediately upon injection. Pain varies from mild to severe and may last for a few minutes or up to 12 hours. Systemic complications of intra-articular corticosteroids are rare; however, mild systemic effects may occur following large doses in multiple joints. Treatment failures are most frequently the result of failure to enter the synovial space. If failures occur when injections into the synovial spaces are certain, as determined by aspiration of fluid, repeated injections are usually futile[126].

REFERENCES

1 Boswell SG, Cole BJ, Sundman EA, *et al.* Platelet-rich plasma: a milieu of bioactive factors. *Arthroscopy* 2012;**28**(3):429–39.

2 Dohan Ehrenfest DM, Doglioli P, de Peppo GM, *et al.* Choukroun's platelet-rich fibrin (PRF) stimulates in vitro proliferation and differentiation of human oral bone mesenchymal stem cell in a dose-dependent way. *Arch Oral Biol* 2010;**55**:185–94.

3 Filardo G, Kon E, Roffi A *et al.* Platelet rich plasma: why intra-articular? A systematic review of preclinical studies and clinical evidence on PRP for joint degeneration. *Knee Surg Sports Traumatol Arthrosc* 2015;**23**(9):2459–74

4 Hsu WK, Mishra A, Rodeo SR, *et al.* Platelet-rich plasma in orthopaedic applications: evidence-based recommendations for treatment. *J Am Acad Orthop Surg* 2013;**21**:739–48.

5 McLellan J, Plevin S. Does it matter which platelet-rich plasma we use? *Equine Vet Educ* 2011;**23**(2):101–4.

6 Pelletier MH, Malhotra A, Brighton T, *et al.* Platelet function and constituents of platelet rich plasma. *Int J Sports Med* 2013;**34**: 74–80.

7 Sundman EA, Cole BJ, Karas V, *et al.* The anti-inflammatory and matrix restorative mechanisms of platelet-rich plasma in osteoarthritis. *Am J Sports Med* 2013;**42**(1): 35–41.

8 Abrams GD, Frank RM, Fortier LA, *et al.* Platelet-rich plasma for articular cartilage repair. *Sports Med Arthrosc Rev* 2013;**21**:213–19.

9 Cho K, Kim JM, Kim MH, *et al.* Scintigraphic evaluation of osseointegrative response around calcium phosphate-coated titanium implants in tibia bone: effect of platelet-rich plasma on bone healing in dogs. *Eur Surg Res* 2013;**51**:138–45.

10 Dragoo JL, Braun HJ, Durham JL, *et al.* Comparison of the acute inflammatory response of two commercial platelet-rich plasma systems in healthy rabbit tendons. *Am J Sports Med* 2012;**40**(6):1274–81.

11 Dragoo JL, Wasterlain AS, Braun HJ, *et al.* Platelet-rich plasma as a treatment for patellar tendinopathy: a double-blind, randomized controlled trial. *Am J Sports Med* 2014;**42**(3):610–18.

12 Filardo G, Kon E, Di Martino A, *et al.* Platelet-rich plasma vs hyaluronic acid to treat knee degenerative pathology: study design and preliminary results of a randomized controlled trial. *BMC Musculoskeletal Disorders* 2012;**13**(229):1–8.

13 Filardo G, Kon E, Buda R, *et al.* Platelet-rich plasma intra-articular knee injections for the treatment of degenerative cartilage lesions and

osteoarthritis. *Knee Surg Sports Traumatol Arthrosc* 2011;**19**:528–35.

14 Franklin S, Cook J. Prospective trial of autologous conditioned plasma versus hyaluronan plus corticosteroid for elbow osteoarthritis in dogs. *Can Vet J* 2013;**54**:881–84.

15 Jang SJ, Kim JD, Cha SS. Platelet-rich plasma (PRP) injections as an effective treatment for early osteoarthritis. *Eur J Orthop Surg Traumatol* 2013;**23**:573–80.

16 Khoshbin A, Leroux T, Wasserstein D, *et al.* The efficacy of platelet-rich plasma in the treatment of symptomatic knee osteoarthritis: a systematic review with quantitative synthesis. *Arthroscopy* 2013;**29**(12):2037–48.

17 Kon E, Buda R, Filardo G, *et al.* Platelet-rich plasma: intra-articular knee injections produced favorable results on degenerative cartilage lesions. *Knee Surg Sports Traumatol Arthrosc* 2010;**18**:474–79.

18 Kon E, Mandelbaum B, Buda R, *et al.* Platelet-rich plasma intra-articular injection versus hyaluronic acid viscosupplementation as treatments for cartilage pathology: from early degeneration to osteoarthritis. *Arthroscopy* 2011;**27**(11):1490–1501.

19 McCarrel T, Fortier L. Temporal growth factor release from platelet-rich plasma, trehalose lyophilized platelets, and bone marrow aspirate and their effect on tendon and ligament gene expression. *J Orthop Res* 2009;**27**(8):1033–42.

20 McCarrel TM, Minas T, Fortier LA. Optimization of leukocyte concentration in platelet-rich plasma for the treatment of tendinopathy. *J Bone Joint Surg Am* 2012;**94**: e143(1–8).

21 Mishra A, Pavelko T. Treatment of chronic elbow tendinosis with buffered platelet-rich plasma. *Am J Sports Med* 2006;**34**(11):1774–78.

22 Patel S, Shillon MS, Aggarwal S, *et al.* Treatment with platelet-rich plasma is more effective than placebo for knee osteoarthritis: a prospective, double-blinded, randomized trial. *Am J Sports Med* 2013;**41**(2):356–64.

23 Raeissadat SA, Rayegani SM, Babaee M, *et al.* The effect of platelet-rich plasma on pain, function, and quality of life of patients with knee osteoarthritis. *Pain Res Treatment* 2013;**1**:1–7.

24 Randelli P, Arrigoni P, Ragone V, *et al.* Platelet rich plasma in arthroscopic rotator cuff repair: a prospective RCT study, 2-year follow-up. *J Shoulder Elbow Surg* 2011;**20**:518–28.

25 Sampson S, Gerhardt M, Mandelbaum B. Platelet rich plasma injection grafts for musculoskeletal injuries: a review. *Curr Rev Musculoskelet Med* 2008;**1**:165–74.

26 Silva RF, Carmona JU, Rezende CMF. Intra-articular injections of autologous platelet concentrates in dogs with surgical reparation of cranial cruciate ligament rupture. *Vet Comp Orthop Traumatol* 2013;**26**:122–25.

27 Smith JJ, Ross MW, Smith RKW. Anabolic effects of acellular bone marrow, platelet rich plasma, and serum on equine suspensory ligament fibroblasts in vitro. *Vet Comp Orthop Traumatol* 2006;**19**:43–7.

28 Souza TFB, Andrade AL, Ferrreira GTNM, *et al.* Healing and expression of growth factors (TGF-B and PDGF) in canine radial osteotomy gap containing platelet-rich plasma. *Vet Comp Orthop Traumatol* 2012;**25**:445–52.

29 Van Buul GM, Koevoet WLM, Kops N, *et al.* Platelet-rich plasma releasate inhibits inflammatory processes in osteoarthritic chondrocytes. *Am J Sports Med* 2011;**39**(11):2362–70.

30 Xie X, Hua W, Zhao S, *et al.* The effect of platelet-rich plasma on patterns of gene expression in a dog model of anterior cruciate ligament reconstruction. *J of Surg Res* 2013;**180**:80–8.

31 Xie X, Wang Y, Zhao C, *et al.* Comparative evaluation of MSCs from bone marrow and adipose tissue seeded in PRP-derived scaffold for cartilage regeneration. *Biomaterials* 2012;**33**:7708–18.

32 Broeckx S, Zimmerman M, Crocetti S, *et al.* Regenerative therapies for equine degenerative joint disease: a preliminary study. *PLoS ONE.* 2014;**9**(1):e85917.

33 Cho HS, Song IH, Park SY, *et al.* Individual variation in growth factor concentrations in platelet-rich plasma and its influence on human mesenchymal stem cells. *Korean J Lab Med* 2011;**31**:212–18.

34 Del Bue M, Riccò S, Ramoni R, *et al.* Equine adipose-tissue derived mesenchymal stem cells and platelet concentrates: their association in vitro and in vivo. *Vet Res Commun* 2008;**32**(S1):S51– S55.

35 Drengk A, Zapf A, Stürmer EK, Stürmer KM, et al. Influence of platelet-rich plasma on chondrogenic differentiation and proliferation of chondrocytes and mesenchymal stem cells. Cells Tissues Organs 2009;189:317–26.

36 Dohan Ehrenfest DM, Rasmusson L, Albrektsson T. Classification of platelet concentrates: from pure platelet-rich plasma (P-PRP) to leukocyte- and platelet-rich fibrin (L-PRF). Trends in Biotech 2008;27(3):158–67.

37 Mishra A, Tummala P, King A, et al. Buffered platelet-rich plasma enhances mesenchymal stem cell proliferation and chondrogenic differentiation. Tissue Eng Part C Methods 2009;15:431–35.

38 Schnabel LV, Lynch ME, Van der Meulen MC, et al. Mesenchymal stem cells and insulin-like growth factor-I gene-enhanced mesenchymal stem cells improve structural aspects of healing in equine flexor digitorum superficialis tendons. J Orthop Res 2009;27(10):1392–98.

39 Torricelli P, Fini M, Filardo G, et al. Regenerative medicine for the treatment of musculoskeletal overuse injuries in competition horses. Internat Orthop 2011;35:1569–76.

40 Braun HJ, Kim HJ, Chu CR, et al. The effect of platelet-rich plasma formulations and blood products on human synoviocytes. Am J Sports Med 2014;42(5):1204–10.

41 Sundman EA, Cole BJ, Fortier LA. Growth factor and catabolic cytokine concentrations are influenced by the cellular composition of platelet-rich plasma. Am J Sports Med 2013;39(10):2135–40.

42 Sundman EA, Boswell SG, Schnabel LV, et al. Increasing platelet concentrations in leukocyte-reduced platelet-rich plasma decrease collagen gene synthesis in tendons. Am J Sports Med 2013;42(1):35–41.

43 Castillo TN, Pouliot MA, Kim HJ, et al. Comparison of growth factor and platelet concentrations from commercial platelet-rich plasma separation systems. Am J Sports Med 2011;39(2):266–71.

44 Stief M, Gottschalk J, Ionita JC, et al. Concentration of platelets and growth factors in canine autologous conditioned plasma. Vet Comp Orthop Traumatol 2011;24:285–90.

45 Boswell SG, Schnabel LV, Mohammed HO, et al. Increasing platelet concentrations in leukocyte-reduced platelet-rich plasma decrease collagen gene synthesis in tendons. Am J Sports Med 2013;42(1):42–9.

46 Cavallo C, Filardo G, Mariani E, et al. Comparison of platelet-rich plasma formulations for cartilage healing. J Bone Joint Surg Am 2014;96:423–29.

47 Naldini A, Morena E, Fimiani M, et al. The effects of autologous platelet gel on inflammatory cytokine response in human peripheral blood mononuclear cells. Platelets 2008;19(4):268–74.

48 Yoshida R, Murray MM. Peripheral blood mononuclear cells enhance the anabolic effects of platelet-rich plasma on anterior cruciate ligament fibroblasts. J Orthop Res 2013;31(1):29–34.

49 Grassel S, Lorenz J. Tissue engineering strategies to repair chondroal and osteochondral tissue in osteoarthritis: use of mesenchymal stem cells. Curr Rheumatol Rep 2014;16:452.

50 Ham O, Lee CY, Kim R, et al. Therapeutic potential of differentiated mesenchymal stem cells for treatment of osteoarthritis. Int J Mol Sci 2015;16:14961–78.

51 Kristjansson B, Honsawek S. Current perspectives in mesenchymal stem cell therapies for osteoarthritis. Stem Cells Int 2014:1–13.

52 Mazor M, Lespessailles E, Coursier R, et al. Mesenchymal stem-cell potential in cartilage repair: an update. J Cell Mol Med 2014;18(12):2340–50.

53 Sampson S, Batto-van Bemden A, Aufiero D. Stem cell therapies for treatment of cartilage and bone disorders: osteoarthritis, avascular necrosis, and non-union fractures. PM R 2015;7:S26–S32.

54 Wang W, Cao W. Treatment of osteoarthritis with mesenchymal stem cells. Sci China Life Sci 2014;57(6):586–95.

55 Wolfstadt JI, Cole BJ, Ogilvie-Harris DJ, et al. Current concepts: the role of mesenchymal stem cells in the management of knee osteoarthritis. Sports Health 2015;7(1):38–44.

56 Kiefer K, Wucherer KL, Pluhar GE, et al. Autologous and allogeneic stem cells as adjuvant therapy for osteoarthritis caused by spontaneous fragmented coronoid process in dogs. In Proceedings VOS Symposium 2013, Canyons Resort, Utah, USA.

57 Cuervo B, Rubio M, Sopena J, et al. Hip osteoarthritis in dogs: a randomized study using

mesenchymal stem cells from adipose tissue and plasma rich in growth factors. *Int J Mol Sci* 2014;**15**:13437–60.

58 Vilar JM, Batista M, Morales M, *et al.* Assessment of th effect of intraarticular injection of autologous adipose derived mesenchymal stem cells in osteoarthritic dogs using a double blinded force platform analysis. *BMC Vet Res* 2014;**10**:143.

59 Vilar JM, Morales M, Santana A, *et al.* Controlled, blinded force platform analysis of the effect of intraarticular injection of autologous adipose-derived mesenchymal stem cells associated to PRGF-Endoret in osteoarthritic dogs. *BMC Vet Res* 2013;**9**:131.

60 Martinello T, Bronzini I, Maccatrozzo L, *et al.* Canine adipose-derived-mesenchymal stem cells do not lose stem features after a long-term cryopreservation. *Res in Veterinary Sci* 2011;**91**:18–24.

61 Carvalho AM, Badial PR, Alvarez LE, *et al.* Equine tendonitis therapy using mesenchymal stem cells and platelet concentrations: a randomized controlled trial. *Stem Cell Res Ther* 2013;**22**(4):85.

62 Ricco S, Renzi S, Del Bue S, *et al.* Allogeneic adipose tissue-derived mesenchymal stem cells in combination with platelet rich plasma are safe and effective in therapy of superficial digital flexor tendonitis in the horse. *Int J Immunopathol Pharmacol* 2013;**26**:61–8.

63 Chen L, Dong SW, Liu JP, *et al.* Synergy of tendon stem cells and platelet-rich-plasma in tendon healing. *J Orthop Res* 2012;**30**(6):991–97.

64 Uysal CA, Tobita M, Hyakusoku H, *et al.* Adipose-derived stem cells enhance primary tendon repair: biomechanical and immunohistochemical evaluation. *J Plast Reconstr Aesthet Surg* 2012;**65**(12):1712–19.

65 Manning CN, Schwartz AG, Liu W, *et al.* Controlled delivery of mesenchymal stem cells and growth factors using a nanofiber scaffold for tendon repair. *Acta Biomater* 2013;**9**(6):6905–14.

66 Yun JH, Han SH, Choi SH, *et al.* Effects of bone marrow-derived mesenchymal stem cells and platelet-rich plasma on bone regeneration for osseointegration of dental implants: preliminary study in canine three-wall intrabony defects. *J Biomed Mater Res B Appl Biomater* 2014;**102**(5):1021–30.

67 Tobita M, Uysal CA, Guo X, *et al.* Periodontal tissue regeneration by combined implantation of adipose tissue-derived stem cells and platelet-rich plasma in a canine model. *Cryotherapy* 2013;**15**(12):1517–26.

68 Astor DE, Hoelzler MG, Harman R, *et al.* Patient factors influencing the concentration of stromal vascular fraction for adipose-derived stromal cell therapy in dogs. *Can Vet J* 2013;**77**(3):177–82.

69 Canapp SO, Carr BJ, Huang R, *et al.* Canine bone marrow aspirate and stromal vascular fraction: prospective analysis. In *Proceedings of ACVS Symposium* 2015. Nashville, TN, USA.

70 Hernigou P, Poignard A, Beaujean F, *et al.* Percutaneous autologous bone-marrow grafting for nonunions: influence of the number and concentration of progenitor cells. *J Bone Joint Surg Am* 2005;**87**A:1430–37.

71 Hauser RA, Eteshola E. Rationale for using direct bone marrow aspirate as a proliferant for regenerative injection therapy. O*pen Stem Cell J* 2013;**4**:7–14.

72 Almaawi A, Wang HT, Cinobanu O, *et al.* Effect of acetaminophen and nonsteroidal anti-inflammatory drugs on gene expression of mesenchymal stem cells. *Tissue Eng Part A* 2013;**19**(7–8):1039–46.

73 Muller M, Raabe O, Addicks K, *et al.* Effects of non-steroidal anti-inflammatory drugs on proliferation, differentiation, and migration in equine mesenchymal stem cells. *Cell Biol Int* 2011;**35**(3):235–48.

74 Salem O, Wang HT, Alaseem A, *et al.* Naproxen affects osteogenesis of human mesenchymal stem cells via regulation of Indian hedgehog signaling molecules. *Arthritis Res Ther* 2014;**16**:R152.

75 Belinski GS, Antic SD. Mild hypothermia inhibits differentiation of human embryonic and induced pluripotent stem cells. *BioTechniques* 2013;**55**:79–82.

76 Heng BC, Cowan CM, Basu S. Temperature and calcium ions affect aggregation of mesenchymal stem cells in phosphate buffered saline. *Cytotechnology* 2008;**58**:69–75.

77 Ginani F, Soares DM, Barreto MP, *et al.* Effect of low-level laser therapy on mesenchymal stem cell proliferation: a systemic review. *Lasers Med Sci* 2015;**30**(8):2189–94.

78 Kushibiki T, Hirasawa T, Okawa S, *et al.* Low reactive laser therapy for mesenchymal stromal cell therapies. *Stem Cell Int* 2015;1–12.

79 Min KH, Byun JH, Heo CY, *et al.* Effect of low-level laser therapy on human adipose-derived stem cells: in vitro and in vivo studies. *Aesth Plast Surg* 2015;**39**:778–82.

80 Park IS, Chung PS, Ahn JC. Enhancement of ischemic wound healing by spheroid grafting of human adipose-derived stem cells treated with low-level light irradiation. *PLOS ONE* 2015;**10**(6):e0122776.

81 Valiati R, Paes JV, de Moraes AN, *et al.* Effect of low-level laser therapy on incorporation of block allografts. 2012;**9**:853–61.

82 Zaccara IM, Ginani F, Moto-Filho HG, *et al.* Effect of low-level laser irradiation on proliferation and viability of human dental pulp stem cells. *Laser Med Sci* 2015;**30**(9):2259–64.

83 Arend WP, Malyak M, Guthridge CJ, *et al.* Interleukin-1 receptor antagonist: role in biology. *Annu Rev Immunol* 1998;**16**:27–55.

84 Arner EC, Harris RR, DiMeo RM, *et al.* Interleukin-1 receptor antagonist inhibits proteoglycan breakdown in antigen induced but not polycation induced arthritis in the rabbit. *J Rheumatol* 1995;**22**(7):1338–46.

85 Bandara G, Meuller GM, Galea-Lauri J, *et al.* Intraarticular expression of biologically active interleukin 1-receptor antagonist protein by ex vivo gene transfer. *Proc Natl Acad Sci USA* 1993;**90**:10764–68.

86 Chen B, Qin J, Wang H, *et al.* Effects of adenovirus-mediated bFGF, IL-1Ra and IGF-1 gene transfer on human osteoarthritic chondrocytes and osteoarthritis in rabbits. *Exper Mol Med* 2010;**42**(10):684–95.

87 Fernandes J, Tardif G, Martel-Pelletier J, *et al.* In vivo transfer of interleukin-1 receptor antagonist gene in osteoarthritic rabbit knee joints. *Am J Path* 1999;**154**(4):1159–69.

88 Frisbie DD, Ghivizzani SC, Robbins PD, *et al.* Treatment of experimental equine osteoarthritis by in vivo delivery of the equine interleukin-1 receptor antagonist gene. *Gene Therapy* 2002;**9**:12–20.

89 Baltzer AWA, Ostapczuk MS, Stosch D, *et al.* A new treatment for hip osteoarthritis: clinical evidence for the efficacy of autologous conditioned serum. *Orthop Rev* 2013;**5**:e13.

90 Bertone AL, Ishihara A, Zekas LJ, *et al.* Evaluation of a single intra-articular injection of autologous protein solution for treatment of osteoarthritis in horses. *Am J Vet Res* 2014;**75**:141–51.

91 Yang KGA, Raijmakers NJH, van Arkel ERA *et al.* Autologous interleukin-1 receptor antagonist improves function and symptoms in osteoarthritis when compared to placebo in a prospective randomized controlled trial. *Osteoarthr Cartilage* 2008;**16**:498–505.

92 Baltzer AW, Moser C, Jansen SA, *et al.* Autologous conditioned serum is an effective treatment for knee osteoarthritis. *Osteoarthritis* 2009;**17**:152–60.

93 Frisbie DD, Kawcak CE, Werpy NM, *et al.* Clinical, biochemical, and histologic effects of intra-articular administration of autologous conditioned serum in horses with experimentally induced osteoarthritis. *Am J Vet Res* 2007;**68**:290–96.

94 Wanstrath A, Hettlich B, Zekas L, *et al.* Intra-articular injection of autologous protein solution for treatment of canine osteoarthritis: a prospective, randomized, double-blinded, placebo-controlled In *Proceedings ACVS Symposium* 2015, Nashville, TN, USA.

95 Meijer H, Reinecke J, Becker C, *et al.* The production of anti-inflammatory cytokines in whole blood by physico-chemical induction. *Inflamm Res* 2003;**52**:404–07.

96 Huggins SS, Suchodolski JS, Bearden RN, *et al.* Serum concentrations of canine interleukin-1 receptor antagonist protein in healthy dogs after incubation using an autologous serum processing system. *Res in Vet Sci* 2015;**101**:28–33.

97 Lussier A, Cividino AA, McFarlane CA, *et al.* Viscosupplementation with hyalgen for the treatment of osteoarthritis: findings from clinical practice in Canada. *J Rheumatol* 1996;**23**:1579–85.

98 Tulamo RM, Heiskanen T, Salonen M. Concentrations and molecular weight distribution of hyaluronate in synovial fluid from clinically normal horses and horses with diseased joints. *Am J Vet Res* 1994;**55**:710–15.

99 Engstrom-Laurent A, Hallgren R. Circulating hyaluronic acid levels vary with physical

activity in healthy subjects and in rheumatoid arthritis patients. Relationship to synovitis mass and morning stiffness. *Arthritis Rheum* 1987;**30**:1333–38.

100 Smith GN, Meyers SL, Brandt KD, *et al.* Effect of intra-articular hyaluronan injection in experimental canine osteoarthritis. *Arthritis Rheum* 1998;**41**:976–85.

101 Budsberg SC, Lenz ME, Thonar EJMA. Serum and synovial fluid concentration of keratan sulfate and hyaluronan in dogs with induced stifle joint osteoarthritis following cranial cruciate ligament transection. *Am J Vet Res* 2006;**67**:429–32.

102 Plickert HD, Bondzio A, Einspanier R, *et al.* Hyaluronic acid concentrations in synovial fluid of dogs with different stages of osteoarthritis. *Res Vet Sci* 2013;**94**:728–34.

103 Band PA, Heeter J, Wisniewski HG, *et al.* Hyaluronan molecular weight distribution is associated with the risk of knee osteoarthritis progression. *Osteoarthr Cartilage* 2015;**23**:70–6.

104 Kuroki K, Cook JL, Kreeger JM. Mechanisms of action and potential use of hyaluronan in dogs with osteoarthritis. *J Am Vet Med Assoc* 2002;**221**(7): 944–50.

105 Smith G, Myers SL, Brandt KD, *et al.* Effect of intraarticular hyaluronan injection on vertical ground reaction force and progression of osteoarthritis after anterior cruciate ligament transection. *J Rhematol* 2005;**32**:325–34.

106 Wang CT, Lin YT, Chiang BL, *et al.* High molecular weight hyaluronic acid down regulates the gene expression of osteoarthritis associated cytokines and enzymes in fibroblast-like synoviocytes from patients with early osteoarthritis. *Osteoarthr Cartil* 2006;**14**:1237–47.

107 Greenberg DD, Stoker A, Kane S, *et al.* Biochemical effects of two different hyaluronic acid products in a co-culture model of osteoarthritis. *Osteoarthr Cartil* 2006;**14**:814–22.

108 Osti L, Berardocco M, di Giacomo V, *et al.* Hyaluronic acid increases tendon derived cell viability and collagen type I expression in vitro: comparative study of four different hyaluronic acid preparations by molecular weight. *BMC Musculoskeletal Disorders* 2015;**16**:284.

109 Altman RD, Schemitsch E, Bedi A. Assessment of clinical practice guideline methodology for the treatment of knee osteoarthritis with intra-articular hyaluronic acid. *Semin Arthritis Rheum* 2015;**45**(2):132–39.

110 Campbell KA, Erickson BJ, Saltzman BM, *et al.* Is local viscosupplementation injection clinically superior to other therapies in the treatment of osteoarthritis of the knee: a systemic review of overlapping meta-analyses. *Arthroscopy* 2015;**31**(10):2036–45.

111 Conrozier T. Optimizing the effectiveness of viscosupplementation in non-knee osteoarthritis. *Joint Bone Spine* 2015;1–2.

112 Henrotin Y, Raman R, Richette P, *et al.* Consensus statement on viscosupplementation with hyaluronic acid for the management of osteoarthritis. *Sem Arthrit Rheum* 2015;1–10.

113 Goldberg VM, Buckwalker JA. Hyaluronans in the treatment of osteoarthritis of the knee: evidence for disease-modifying activity. *Osteoarthr Cartilage* 2005;**13**:216–24.

114 Schiavinato A, Lini E, Guidolin D, *et al.* Intraarticular sodium hyaluronate injections in the Pond-Nuki experimental model of osteoarthritis in dogs. II. Morphological findings. *Clin Orthop Relat Res* 1989;**241**:286–99.

115 Smith GN, Mickler EA, Myers SL. Effect of intra-articular hyaluronan injection on synovial fluid hyaluronan in the early stage of canine post-traumatic osteoarthritis. *J Rheumatol* 2001;**28**:1341–46.

116 Marshall KW. Viscosupplementation for osteoarthritis: current status, unresolved issues, and future directions. *J Rheumatol* 1998;**25**(11):2056–58.

117 Iannitti T, Elhensheri M, Bingol AO, *et al.* Preliminary histopathological study of intra-articular injection of novel highly cross-linked hyaluronic acid in a rabbit model of knee osteoarthritis. *J Mol Histol* 2013;**44**(2):191–201.

118 Marshall KW, Manolopoulos V, Mancer K, *et al.* Amelioration of disease severity by intraarticular hylan therapy in bilateral canine osteoarthritis. *J Orthop Res* 2000;**18**(3):416–25.

119 Petrella RJ, Petrella M. A prospective, randomized, double-blind, placebo controlled study to evaluate the efficacy of intraarticular hyaluronic acid for osteoarthritis of the knee. *J Rheumatol* 2006;**33**(5):951–56.

120 Kotevoglu N, Iyibozkurt PC, Hiz O, *et al.* A prospective randomized controlled clinical trial comparing the efficacy of different molecular weight hyaluronan solutions in the treatment of knee osteoarthritis. *Rheumatol Int* 2006;**26**(4):325–30.

121 Reichenbach S, Blank S, Rutjes AW, *et al.* Hylan versus hyaluronic acid for osteoarthritis of the knee: a systemic review and meta-analysis. *Arthritis Rheum* 2007;**57**(8):1410–18.

122 Hellstrom LE, Carlsson C, Boucher JF, *et al.* Intra-articular injections with high molecular weight sodium hyaluronate as therapy for canine arthritis. *Vet Rec* 2003;**153**:89–90.

123 Pelletier JP, Mineau F, *et al.* Intraarticular injections with methylprednisolone acetate reduce osteoarthritic lesions in parallel with chondrocyte stromelysis synthesis in experimental osteoarthritis. *Arthritis Rheum* 1994;**37**(3):414–23.

124 Sherman SL, Khazai RS, James CH, *et al.* In vitro toxicity of local anesthetics and corticosteroids on chondrocyte and synoviocyte viability and metabolism. *Cartilage* 2015;**6**(4):233–40.

125 Cole BJ, Schumacher HR Jr. Injectable corticosteroids in modern practice. *J Am Acad Orthop Surg* 2005;**13**(1):37–46.

126 Tynjala P, Honkanen V, Lahdenne P. Intra-articular steroids in radiologically confirmed tarsal and hip synovitis of juvenile idiopathic arthritis. *Clin and Exper Rheum* 2004;**22**:643–48.

127 Bakker AC, van de Loo FA, van Beuningen HM, *et al.* Overexpression of active TGF-beta-1 in the murine knee joint: evidence for synovial-layer-dependent chondro-osteophyte formation. *Osteoarthr Cartilage* 2001;**9**:128–36.

128 Baltzer AW, Moser C, Jansen SA, *et al.* Autologous conditioned serum (Orthokine) is an effective treatment for knee osteoarthritis. *Osteoarthr Cartilage* 2009;**17**:152–60.

129 Elshaier AM, Hakimiyan AA, Rappoport L, *et al.* Effect of interleukin-1beta on osteogenic protein1-induced signaling in adult human articular chondrocytes. *Arthritis Rheum* 2009;**60**:143–54.

130 Irrgang JJ, Anderson AF, Boland AL *et al.* Development and validation of the International Knee Documentation Committee subjective knee form. *Am J Sports Med* 2001;**29**:600–13.

131 Sun Y, Feng Y, Zhang CQ, *et al.* The regenerative effect of platelet-rich plasma on healing in large osteochondral defects. *Int Orthop* 2010;**34**:589–97.

132 Wakitani S, Saito T, Caplan AI. Myogenic cells derived from rat bone marrow mesenchymal stem cells exposed to 5-azacytidine. *Muscle Nerve* 1995;**18**:1417–26.

133 Blaney Davidson EN, van der Kraan PM, van den Berg WB. TGF-beta and osteoarthritis. *Osteoarthr Cartilage* 2007;**15**:597–604.

134 Wakitani S, Saito T, Caplan AI. Myogenic cells derived from rat bone marrow mesenchymal stem cells exposed to 5-azacytidine. *Muscle Nerve* 1995;**18**:1417–26.

135 Badlani N, Inoue A, Healey R, *et al.* The protective effect of OP-1 on articular cartilage in the development of osteoarthritis. *Osteoarthr Cartilage* 2008;**16**:600–606.

136 Goodrich LR, Hidaka C, Robbins PD, *et al.* Genetic modification of chondrocytes with insulin-like growth factor-1 enhances cartilage healing in an equine model. *J Bone Joint Surg Br* 2007;**89**:672–85.

137 Miller Y, Bachowski G, Benjamin R, *et al. Practice Guidelines for Blood Transfusion: A Compilation From Recent Peer-reviewed Literature.* 2nd ed. Washington, DC: American Red Cross; 2007:56.

138 Schmidt MB, Chen EH, Lynch SE. A review of the effects of insulin-like growth factor and platelet derived growth factor on in vivo cartilage healing and repair. *Osteoarthr Cartilage* 2006;**14**:403–12.

139 Schnabel LV, Mohammed HO, Miller BJ, *et al.* Platelet rich plasma (PRP) enhances anabolic gene expression patterns in flexor digitorum superficialis tendons. J *Orthop Res* 2007;**25**:230–40.

140 Fan H, Tao H, Wu Y, *et al.* TGF-b3 immobilized PLGA-gelatin/chondroitin sulfate/hyaluronic acid hybrid scaffold for cartilage regeneration. *J Biomed Mater Res A* 2010;**95**:982–92.

141 Lee SH, Shin H. Matrices and scaffolds for delivery of bioactive molecules in bone and cartilage tissue engineering. *Adv Drug Deliv Rev* 2007;**59**:339–59.

142 Miyakoshi N, Kobayashi M, Nozaka K, *et al.* Effects of intraarticular administration of basic fibroblast growth factor with hyaluronic acid on osteochondral defects of the knee in rabbits. *Arch Orthop Trauma Surg* 2005;**125**:683–92.

143 Wu MY, Hill CS. TGF-beta superfamily signaling in

embryonic development and homeostasis. *Dev Cell* 2009;**16**:329–43.

144 Ekenstedt KJ, Sonntag WE, Loeser RF, *et al.* Effects of chronic growth hormone and insulin-like growth factor 1 deficiency on osteoarthritis severity in rat knee joints *Arthritis Rheum* 2006;**54**:3850–58.

145 Gouttenoire J, Valcourt U, Ronziere MC, *et al.* Modulation of collagen synthesis in normal and osteoarthritic cartilage. *Biorheology* 2004;**41**:535–42.

146 Middleton J, Manthey A, Tyler J. Insulin-like growth factor (IGF) receptor, IGF-I, interleukin-1b (IL-1b), and IL-6 mRNA expression in osteoarthritic and normal human cartilage. *J Histochem Cytochem* 1996;**44**:133–41.

147 Smyth SS, McEver RP, Weyrich AS, *et al.* Platelet Colloquium Participants. Platelet functions beyond hemostasis. *J Thromb Haemost* 2009;**7**:1759–66.

148 Ellman MB, An HS, Muddasani P, *et al.* Biological impact of the fibroblast growth factor family on articular cartilage and intervertebral disc homeostasis. *Gene* 2008;**420**:82–9.

149 Mishra A, Tummala P, King A, *et al.* Buffered platelet-rich plasma enhances mesenchymal stem cell proliferation and chondrogenic differentiation. *Tissue Eng Part C Methods* 2009;**15**:431–35.

150 Hayashi M, Muneta T, Ju YJ, *et al.* Weekly intra-articular injections of bone morphogenetic protein-7 inhibits osteoarthritis progression. *Arthritis Res Ther* 2008;**10**:R118.

151 Maehara H, Sotome S, Yoshii T, *et al.* Repair of large osteochondral defects in rabbits using porous hydroxyapatite/collagen (HAp/Col) and fibroblast growth factor-2 (FGF-2). *J Orthop Res* 2010;**28**:677–86.

Note: page numbers in *italics* refer to figures and tables.